D0389132

ELEGY FOR A DISEASE

ELEGY FOR A DISEASE

A Personal and Cultural History of Polio

ANNE FINGER

ST. MARTIN'S PRESS NEW YORK

The names and identifying characteristics of some individuals depicted in the book have been changed.

www.stmartins.com

Library of Congress Cataloging-in-Publication Data

Finger, Anne.
    Elegy for a disease : a personal and cultural history of polio / Anne Finger.—
1st ed.
      p. cm.
    ISBN-13: 978-0-312-34757-4
    ISBN-10: 0-312-34757-X
    1. Finger, Anne. 2. Finger, Anne—Health. 3. Poliomyelitis—Patients—
Michigan—Biography. 4. Poliomyelitis—United States—History—20th century.
  5. Poliomyelitis—Social aspects—United States—History—20th century. I. Title

RC180.2.F56 2006
362.196'835—dc22
[B]
                                              2006047660

First Edition: November 2006

10 9 8 7 6 5 4 3 2 1

For Karen

ACKNOWLEDGMENTS

My deep thanks to Max Finger, Simi Linton, Brian Thorstenson, Stephen Pelton, Karen Donovan, Susan Finger, Margo Wechsler, and Susan Roth, who not only have been wonderful friends but have read drafts of the book and given me invaluable help along the way. In addition, Susan Finger was enormously helpful with research assistance. Steve Taylor's assistance with information about state institutions for people with developmental disabilities was generous and timely. I owe a special debt of gratitude to Stephen Pelton and Judy Green for urging me to write honestly about difficult periods of my life.

This book would not have been possible without the disability-rights movement and the field of disability studies that has grown from it. I cannot possibly include everyone from that world who has nurtured and sustained me, challenged me, and filled me with hope and laughter, but I would be remiss indeed if I didn't name John Belluso, Gene Chelberg, Kenny Fries, Lakshmi Fjord, Rosemarie Garland-Thomson, Carol Gill, Jenny Kern, Georgina Kleege, Cathy Kudlick, Victoria Lewis, Simi Linton, Paul Longmore, Marsha Saxton, Corbett O'Toole, Alice Sheppard, Sue Schweik, and Barbara Waxman.

I'm deeply grateful to those who were willing to share their knowledge and experiences with me, often of intimate and painful parts of their pasts. A special thanks to Larry Kohout and Henry Haverstock.

Enormous thanks to my wonderful agent, Nat Sobel, and everyone at St. Martin's, especially my editor, Diane Reverand.

Finally, Nomad Cafe and Bittersweet Café kept me caffeinated and provided me with a change of scene from the room of my own.

The microbe is nothing; the terrain is everything.

—LOUIS PASTEUR

I was physically disabled, and no one who hasn't lived the life of a semi-cripple knows how much that means. I think it perhaps was the most important thing that happened to me, and formed me, guided me, instructed me, helped me, and humiliated me—all those things at once. I have never gotten over it, and I am aware of the force and power of it.

—DOROTHEA LANGE

ELEGY FOR
A DISEASE

THE THING ITSELF

In high school I turned the page in my chemistry book, and there before me was a photograph of the molecules of the polio virus. Taken through an electron microscope, the picture could have been faked by setting fifteen or twenty Ping-Pong balls next to one another and snapping a picture of them in a dim room with black-and-white film well past its expiration date.

The photograph evoked a vertiginous feeling in me: How could the thing that had so radically altered my life be so simple?

THE KID IN THE PARKING LOT OF
WAREHOUSE CLUB

I'm exhausted when I limp out of Warehouse Club, a discount supermarket on the outskirts of Detroit, where cartons have been razor-bladed open to reveal their contents: ten-pound sacks of rice or half a dozen boxes of tissues shrink-wrapped together. My cart is loaded down with industrial-size quantities of toilet paper and breakfast cereal and cans of tuna.

One of the neighborhood kids who hang around the doors asks me if I want help. Instead of my usual "No thanks, I'm okay," I let him help me. It's partly that I'm beat, but also that I'm doing him a good turn as much as he's doing me one.

"What happened to your leg?" he asks me as he's loading the groceries into the trunk of my Volvo.

"I had polio."

"What's that?"

I feel like an aging movie star who's been asked her name by a restaurant maître d'. Polio was as famous as AIDS. Those of us who had it were *figures*. We limped around under its metaphoric weight. Polio had such cachet that occasionally people lied and said they had it when they hadn't. Having "overcome" polio was something you could put on life's résumé.

"It's a disease. People don't get it anymore. There's a vaccine now," I say, and hand him two dollars.

"Thanks, lady," he says.

THE BARE BONES OF AN ANSWER

How do I go beyond the bare-bones answer: "It's a disease. People don't get it anymore. There's a vaccine now"?

Since medicine has so often been put at the center of discussions about illness and disability, a medical definition may seem like a logical place to begin: "Poliomyelitis is a common, acute viral disease characterized clinically by a brief febrile illness with sore throat, headache and vomiting, and often with stiffness of the neck and back. In many cases a lower neuron paralysis develops in the early days of illness."

In those sentences a human being is present only by inference. Surely it is a person who experiences the fever—who feels her body being clothed in a thin garment of sweat, who is aware of her urine's heat as it flows from her body. Surely there is someone whose head aches, whose neck seems to move like a rusty hinge. And surely someone who experiences that last symptom—paralysis: not the neat deadness so often assumed to be the lot of the paralytic but a state ripe with paradoxes.

With polio the body is not silent, as it is when the paralysis is a result of spinal cord injury. Anesthesia, absence of feeling, does not accompany polio paralysis because the virus attacks the motor neurons, leaving the nerves that carry sensation intact. In fact, just the opposite of deadening occurs: The affected parts of the body may be more sensitive, nerves jangling and twittering, so that touch itself can become painful. Some parts of my right leg are as acutely sensitive as my clitoris.

Viral infection has a haphazard quality, unlike most spinal cord injury, where the cord is severed ("I'm a C-7," my friends say, or "an L-6," naming the exact vertebra, cervical, thoracic, or lumbar; made even neater in common parlance—"paralyzed from the neck down," "paralyzed from the waist down"—rendering away all function and sensation controlled by the nerves below that vertebra.) My right leg, below my knee, is incapable of any movement save one: I can squeeze my toes downward. I have some very limited function in my right quadriceps—seated, I can lift my leg a couple of inches above the floor. On the inside of my thigh there's a muscle I can flex—trying to find the words to name it, I go on the Internet and find a site that gives a multicolored line drawing of the muscles of a leg along with their Latin names, but I can't figure out which of those is the lonely muscle I can tighten and release, an island of function marooned in a sea of paralysis.

In this story of polio the bodies of those who experience the illness will be present, but not just our bodies. Polio, a physical experience, is also a social one. The historian Charles E. Rosenberg noted: "Disease serves as a structuring factor in social situations, as a social actor and mediator. This is an ancient truth. It would hardly have surprised a leper in the twelfth century, or a plague victim in the fourteenth."

It is not just those who have a disease who understand this ancient truth. Polio belongs not just to those of us who were paralyzed by it but to our mothers and fathers, our sisters and brothers, our partners and our children; to those who cared for us, to those who brutalized us—not mutually exclusive categories; to those who saw us as palimpsests on which to write their discomfort, their fear, their pity, their admiration, their empathy.

Polio's meanings change over time: In one era it was an unnamed affliction; in another, it was a disease linked to the "immigrant menace"; during the Depression, the disease that had supposedly disabled Roosevelt and that he had famously "overcome" became emblematic of the grit and determination with which our nation would rise from its economic paralysis. Later it became a symbol of the power of technology to solve our ills. The story of polio became the story of its conquest. Now it is so unknown to a younger generation of Americans that people under thirty sometimes transmute the strange word into a familiar one, "polo"— which causes no end of merriment on our part. "Quite a whack you got from that mallet." "Actually, it was an allergic reaction—too much Ralph Lauren cologne."

THE STORIES I'M NOT GOING TO TELL

I'm not going to tell the story of the plucky little cripple stepping gamely forward on two wooden crutches—if she's a girl, her hair is in Shirley Temple curls and she's wearing a pale blue dress with smocking across the bodice and puff sleeves; if he's a boy, he has a cowlick, wears a cowboy hat, and has a toy silver sheriff's badge pinned to his shirt: those heartbreaking kids, frozen for all time on a March of Dimes poster.

This won't be the elegiac story with its expected arc beginning with normalcy—buckteeth, swimming, football, swings in maple trees, sprinklers whipping across suburban lawns—and then ascending into crisis—dizzying weakness, iron lungs, hot packs with their cloying smell of wet wool, the Dalíesque landscape of high fever; after that the slow and painful resolution of rehabilitation—"Every day another muscle, and on to Berlin in the morning," as Wilfred Sheed, author and polio survivor, put it. And then the hard-won ending, with its return to the empire of the normal, albeit in a wounded body; the final chapters of the narrative, when not just the body but the self has been chastened, and from that chastening, grown.

If I tried to fit my life story into that narrative framework, the main event of my life would have occurred before I reached the age of three, and all the decades since would have been nothing but slow denouement. But that is not the primary reason I reject that way of telling this story.

I do not want to give you just my story. It is not only that I've grown tired of the solipsistic tendencies of contemporary American writing—

although that is true—but also that I want to write about the social experience of disability, not just the personal. In literature disability has most often served as a metaphor. We need only think of Captain Hook and Captain Ahab and Long John Silver—all these characters springing to mind without our even having touched dry land—men whose evil, desire for vengeance, and general air of nefariousness are all hung upon a missing limb. Autobiographical works—including recent memoirs by Nancy Mairs, Leonard Kriegel, Kenny Fries, and Steve Kuusisto—provide an antidote to such neat formulations, presenting the lives of disabled people in their complexity and variety.

And yet autobiography—especially in its reception by an audience already expecting the arc of the story to be that of a singular disabled person, struggling against the constraints of his or her impairment—has the drawback of re-creating the notion of disability as an individual issue, one that will be solved by that person's adjustment to a set of straitened circumstances. In this memoir I will talk about my own experience of polio but will do so against a background of social experiences of the disease, which structure the nondisabled as well as the disabled.

How deeply rooted is the expectation that disabled people should be alone, separated from others, even if we are no longer segregated in institutions? Not long ago I was in a writing workshop at which I was the only disabled person. A photographer, writing an autobiographical text to accompany her photographs, showed a picture she had taken of an armless street seller in India. We had quite a conversation about this photograph, as she explained that she had become a Buddhist after taking this picture. When I asked why, she said: "Don't you see? He has no arms! "Yes," I said, "I see that—but what was the connection between that and your religious conversion?" She could only repeat, as if explaining something to a very dense child—"Don't you see? He has no arms!" And furthermore she said she knew—when I asked how, she said she *just knew*—that his parents had cut off his arms to make him a better beggar: People in India did things like that.

And then she said that the picture had originally included another, nondisabled street seller—someone who leaned over and made change for the man without arms.

I asked her how she had made the decision to crop him out—but before she could answer, several other voices from around the table chimed in: "Oh, I like the picture better with just him." "It's a stronger picture this way." All this without having ever seen the uncropped photo.

The notion that disabled people should be alone, isolated, not in community with others, is so deeply entrenched that we *know* the picture is a better picture with him on his own. We know it without ever having seen the other photograph. Those enormous institutions housing disabled people that once dotted the landscape may have been shut down, but much of that habit of segregation still persists—a need to isolate, to contain, to keep the disabled body from contaminating the normal. "Just him," the voices chorus from around the workshop table. "Him alone," chanting a prejudice they do not even know they have absorbed.

In conventional photographs of disabled people our bodies are nearly always solitary. We stare into the camera, immobilized, our "defects" displayed. Whatever the story of our life was, it is over. The narrative has happened. Our bodies are ruins. The viewer no more asks what will happen next than the traveler gazing at the Pantheon or the Colosseum wonders about its future, other than to hope it will remain forever unchanged. We are the final scene, the aftermath.

Before the conversation about the armless street seller, I'd seen a picture by Sebastião Salgado in the *New York Times*. I stashed the folded-up section of the paper in my canvas tote bag. All that day I kept pulling it out to show friends, calling people and saying, "Do you get the *Times*? . . . Look at the picture on page four in the Science Section. . . . Isn't it wonderful?"

Outside a school in New Delhi, India, children, nearly all of whom have had polio, the caption tells us, are shown. About a dozen of them are seated on a bench—a few look withdrawn, one or two have their backs to the camera—but the rest are horsing around, laughing. We can imagine all kinds of futures for these kids. The pensive boy in the background will grow up to be a poet—or perhaps a software engineer. The laughing girl at the center of the photo, grabbing her friend's nose, will become a theater director or a professor of literature, who lectures to packed classrooms and always has a line of students outside her office door. Perhaps the girl with her back to the camera is the rival of the one with her hair in braids; perhaps the unseen expression on her face is saying to her coterie behind her: *Bharati is so childish!* with all the righteousness about maturity a twelve-year-old can muster. Whatever their stories are, they are not over, and they are not alone.

Within the disability-rights movement—and the academic field of disability studies, which exists in a symbiotic relationship to it—we rarely think in diagnostic categories. We focus instead on social perceptions and barriers to access, the richness of the lived experience of disability. In this book I turn the lens of disability studies on a particular disease, for individual diseases do have meanings, biographies, histories. I explore how the character of polio was cobbled together by hundreds of thousands of acts, ways of speaking, historical accidents, economic forces, acts of resistance. It was shaped by the medicine, by those disabled by it, by those who feared it.

A History of Poliomyelitis—from which I took the medical definition a few pages back—was written by a doctor, and so I suppose I should not be surprised that out of the more than fifty illustrations and photographs in the book, only two depict a person with polio. One is a photograph of an Egyptian grave marker showing a priest with a withered leg—the earliest representation of polio. The other is an anonymous man with his head sticking out of an iron lung—and I suppose I shouldn't be surprised that the caption does not even note the presence of the patient, describing what is shown above as "An early model of the Drinker Respirator known as the 'iron lung.' " (When respiratory muscles were paralyzed, an iron lung was used as a mechanical replacement.)

There's a portrait of Michael Underwood (1738–circa 1810), reputed to be the first physician to have written about polio, his face half shadowed beneath a powdered wig; an obviously posed photograph of Rudolf Virchow (1821–1902), the German pathologist, studying a slide through a magnifying glass. The photographic portraits of Simon Flexner, Ivar Wickman, David Bodian—the great men of the battle against polio—could equally well be bank presidents or professors in the classics department of Ivy League universities. Some others are posed, in white coats, near microscopes or other laboratory paraphernalia.

The story follows the pattern of fairy tales in which suitor after suitor vies unsuccessfully for the hand of the beautiful princess. In this case a dragon need not be slain or a series of trials undergone so that true love can be proved; instead a vaccine must be found to prevent the disease. As it should be in such stories, the victor is from a humble background. In this case not a woodcutter from a cottage on the edge of the forest, but the son of Russian Jewish immigrant parents.

I should not be surprised that when a doctor writes the history, doctors and scientists are given center stage. Utopians begin by looking in the mirror, and I suppose historians do too.

A SLIVER OF TIME

Some of us—in the industrialized world or in countries where there was socialized medicine—lived during a brief sliver of time unique in human history: We lived without the threat of serious epidemic disease, a time during which the U.S. surgeon general could tell Congress, with what now seems like almost laughable naïveté, "We can now close the book on infectious diseases."

That sliver of time began on April 12, 1955, when church bells all across the United States rang. Handwritten signs appeared in the windows of butcher shops and haberdashers and beauty salons that read THANK YOU, DR. SALK.

I know this because I've read it in books. I was three and a half years old on that day, and so I remember nothing of it—although I do remember my trip home from the hospital two months before. My father had told me that my sister Susan was downstairs in the car, waiting for us, sitting behind the steering wheel. I thought that the steering wheel must be one of the four wheels of the car, and I imagined my sister Susan crouched on the ground underneath the car. The "Susan" I imagined was a platonic ideal of a sister. Since I had not seen any of my sisters for six months, they had become creatures simultaneously vague and mythic. I had only glimpsed my brother, born six weeks after I contracted polio, from a hospital window, as my grandparents held him up for me to see. Later, when we drove home, we ate graham crackers, and I thought the golden flecks on Susan's tweed coat were graham cracker crumbs.

And then another flash of memory from one of the official days in my family's calendar, The Day I Came Home from the Hospital. I'm leaning on my wooden underarm crutches in the kitchen, my sister Jane staring up at me. The look on her face is puzzled, and I am looking at her just as quizzically. Both of us seem to be saying to ourselves, *Is this the sister I have heard so much about?* In the memory Jane is wearing glasses—but can that be right? After all, she'd just turned two. It was Sandra who wore glasses then. So maybe I've grafted together my memories of Sandra and Jane, created a composite figure.

I have to fight to keep the face of the Jane I know today from washing over the child's face—although there is a way she has of cocking her head, giving a half smile, that has persisted through the decades. Is the expression I remember on her face really from that day? Or is it from a photograph of all five of us taken a few months later, a photograph I've looked at again and again? In that picture my off-camera mother must have said, "Smile!" and we didn't just smile, we started giggling, one of those wild fits of girl giggles that would sometimes come upon us four sisters. Jane is the one in the photograph who isn't guffawing, sitting with her head bent slightly to the right, that same puzzled look on her face. But the feeling from that flash of memory, that day in the kitchen, is right: the shock of what should be familiar colliding with my sense of utter strangeness. I am not sure of anything else, but I am sure of that sense of emotional vertigo. That I remember.

No, I don't remember that day, April 12, 1955, but I can imagine that in our old farmhouse with sloping floors on East Lake Moraine Road—about a mile outside downtown Hamilton, New York (downtown: a five-and-dime, a Rexall drugstore, a bank, an inn, a stoplight)—we would have been close enough to hear bells ringing in the town's four churches, Catholic, Episcopal, Baptist, and Methodist. Perhaps our black telephone rang, Mrs. Blum or Mrs. Brown or Mrs. Sio—mothers were not Lisa or Debby or Kathleen in those days—calling to tell my mother the news. Or perhaps those women, doing housework—not in black leggings or jeans and baggy T-shirts but in red lipstick and dresses with cinched waists, wearing low-heeled pumps or loafers—hearing the news coming over their substantial radios, had gone over to their black telephones with the heavy receivers—nearly all telephones were black and immovable then, and they never got lost. It was quite unimaginable that one day my mother's raft of daughters would ourselves be mothers, who would stalk around our living rooms muttering, "What did I do with that goddamn telephone?" Perhaps those mothers picked up those telephone receivers to call my mother—and then stood there, with their hand on the telephone, while the operator's voice crackled into the air, "Number, please? Number, please?" Perhaps they would have thought better of it, said, "Never mind. I'm sorry to have—" before they replaced the receiver in its cradle.

And, on the other side of that sliver of time without epidemic disease? There was no such defining moment. I know I glanced at stories in the free weeklies aimed at the gay community in San Francisco, where my partner, Mark, and I were living then. Four or five gay men had died in Los Angeles and New York of a particularly virulent pneumonia. Then more people were dying, and the stories started to move to the front pages. Then they were appearing in the *San Francisco Chronicle*.

While I was writing this I considered going to the library in San Francisco and getting copies of those articles. I decided, though, that I wanted to leave my memories as I remember them: those days when the disease seemed something sad but remote. It was background noise—sirens in the night, voices giving the rush-hour traffic reports on the radio, "A pretty serious accident on the Army Street off-ramp in San Francisco has traffic backed up through . . ." It was drowned out by things that were closer to me: a fight with Mark, a political struggle within the women's group I was part of.

And then, of course, the noises kept coming closer, no longer background.

One evening, when I was living in Detroit, my phone rang. A voice I didn't recognize asked, "Is this Anne Finger?" She told me her name—I don't remember it now—saying she was Jeff Goodman's cousin. Jeff had lived upstairs from me in Venice, California. I thought the next thing she was going to say was: I'm moving to Detroit, Jeff gave me your name, maybe we could have lunch sometime.

Instead she said, "I'm calling to tell you that Jeff died on Wednesday. His funeral's going to be—"

A sound came out of my chest, the sort of cowlike moan I made when I was in labor.

Then I screamed: "No! No! I didn't know he was sick. I didn't even know he was sick."

I was furious at her. I hated her.

"I'm so sorry," she said. "I thought you knew. You were on the list of people to call about the funeral—"

"I didn't know!"

"I thought you knew," she said again. "You were on the list he left of people to call about the funeral."

I moaned the word "Oh."

"I wouldn't have told you like that. I thought you knew."

I didn't hate her anymore. I loved her, momentarily, ferociously.

"Was it AIDS?"

"Yes," she said. Then she said again, "I thought you knew. I wouldn't have told you that way." Then she started to give me details about the funeral.

"Wait a minute, let me get a pen." On a scrap of paper I scratched a date, a time, a place.

For weeks after I came back from his funeral in Los Angeles, a voice in my head kept repeating: *I don't understand why this happened. This doesn't make any sense.*

How did I become this person, how did we become these people, for whom death was supposed to make sense? Why did we think a disease should have its reasons?

A few years later I was at my sister's house in Seattle. It was a Sunday afternoon, and she was groggy, having just woken up from a nap.

"Anne Vanderslice called. To tell you someone died." She yawned, said, "Sorry. I can't remember his name. He worked at Modern Times."

I knew it must be Tede, and I knew he must have died of AIDS. Even though I knew that, I hoped it was someone else, or that he at least got hit by a truck. I knew he would be just as dead, but still it would be a relief to me if it were something besides AIDS. I just couldn't stand to have it be the same thing, over and over and over and over again.

"Tede?"

"Yes."

"AIDS?"

"Yes."

Later that day, my son, Max, and I were sitting in a café when I sighed, and he said, "Are you feeling sad about your friend?" He knew that sigh. He had grown up with this; he thought it was just part of the way the world worked, that every couple of months someone I loved disappeared from the earth.

When Max was six, I took him and a few of his friends to see a movie in which two kids pricked their fingers and rubbed their blood together to become blood sister and blood brother. Driving home, I rehearsed what I was going to say carefully, so it would sound important without being frightening. "Those two children rubbed their blood together, but you shouldn't ever—"

A chorus of "Uh-*duhhh*, H-I-V," rose from the backseat of my old Volvo. We had gone back to living as humanity had always lived, our lives shadowed by the reality of this epidemic, the possibility of more.

Polio isn't the only epidemic disease that shaped my life. My great-great-great-grandfather, Michael Donovan, and great-great-great-grandmother—her name, like the names of so many women, is unknown—left county Cork in 1848, during the potato famine, bound for Halifax, Nova Scotia. They had at least one child with them, Dennis Donovan, then seven years of age. On board one of those ships leaving Ireland, so crowded and thick with disease they were known as coffin ships, Michael and his wife contracted ship fever, or typhus. They reached the promised land only to die.

I suppose one could say they died of natural causes. On the other hand, typhus becomes epidemic when hungry people are crowded together. It runs rampant in jails and concentration camps, during famines and wars, so one could say that the cause of typhus is not so much *Rickettsia prowazekii*, the bacterium causing the disease, as it is social dislocation and oppression. Then again, if it hadn't been for the fungus *Phytophthora infestans*, which blighted the potatoes, Michael Donovan and his family would never have crowded into the steerage of a teeming ship and sailed across the cold, cold Atlantic. But was blight the real cause of the famine? During the famine years Ireland was exporting food— more than enough to feed its population. It wasn't a lack of food but a market economy that caused starvation. As in any epidemic, the natural and the social twist together, a skein of yarn so tangled its threads are impossible to tease free.

What was my great-great-great-grandmother's name? Bridget? Cathleen? Mary? Was my great-great-great-grandmother just a few years removed from being a girl herself? Was she amazed at this son she had given birth to? Or had she given birth to a brood of children, was she worn down and dour, was the famine one more blow in a life filled with them? Had she lost her children one by one during those last years of the 1840s? Or did they survive only to die aboard ship? Or were the sisters and brothers separated from one another in the New World? And what about Dennis, after his parents died? He must have been quarantined. I try to imagine him, in whatever makeshift camp he was held, wondering if he, too, would sicken and die? Did some mother who'd lost her own children latch onto him, the two of them clinging to each other, each one filling for the other the abyss of loss?

I like to imagine that when he was taken it was by a childless couple who heard about these Irish orphans, washed ashore like treasures from a shipwreck. Good Protestants, surely, because later Dennis Donovan became a Baptist minister—as did his son, my great-grandfather, who every year wrote a letter to the Peterborough, New Hampshire, school board, urging them to abandon the licentious practice of holding square dances for the high school students. Maybe the upright Halifax family that took him in saw a soul in danger of perdition—a papish idolater, a worshipper of stocks and stones—and were determined to scourge his wayward soul. Maybe they brought little Dennis home and eased him into a featherbed, gave him a glass of milk still warm from the cow, a slice of bread hot from the oven. I know that isn't likely—records of Irish orphans list them at the age of two as destitute, at the age of five as servants. Or maybe nobody came for him; maybe he went to an orphanage. What legacies of loss and shame and guilt were passed down to me, handed down to my mother and then from my mother to me, along with my blue eyes and stubby fingers?

A reference book entitled *The Encyclopedia of Plague and Pestilence* begins with an entry for "Afghan Cholera Epidemics in the 1930s and 1940s" and ends with "Zanzibar Cholera Epidemic of 1869." In between is information about a few exotic-sounding diseases: Kyasanur Forest Disease of Southern India, a tick-borne virus belonging to the Russian spring-summer viruses; Dancing Mania, also known as St. John's Dance,

St. Vitus's Dance, tarantism, which may have been episodes of mass hysteria, or may also have been caused by rye bread infected with ergot; and epidemics afflicting the Crusader armies at Acre, Adalia, Al Mansurah, Antioch, and Damietta. Before long the book becomes monotonous: epidemics of cholera, smallpox, meningitis, malaria, dysentery, plague, typhus, yellow fever, measles, poliomyelitis, on one page breaking out in Sydney, on another in Samoa. In the 1931 U.S. polio epidemic, 4,138 people died; the Venice plague of 1575–77 killed some fifty thousand; a mid-seventeenth-century outbreak of measles decimated the Huron Indian nation.

Some even think that roughly a million years ago, in the African forests, a viral epidemic like polio or meningitis left protohumans too weak to swing through the branches, and the survivors, eking out an existence on the ground, launched our species.

"SHE'LL BE THREE AT THE END OF OCTOBER"

Prehistory refers to times preceding the beginning of the written record, prior to Herodotus's writing of Xerxes' Persian army marching into Greece, of Thucydides' accounts of the Athenian armies battling the Spartans, or of Ssu-ma Ch'ien's writings on the Chinese courts. History begins when accounts are written, facts are set down.

We know the prehistoric past by supposition and inference, what we extrapolate from myths, what we learn from the archaeological fragments extracted from the earth.

All of us have our own prehistories: our early childhoods.

In the late summer and very early fall of 1954, in the college town of Hamilton in the dairy country of upstate New York, my mother must have answered questions about my age by saying, "She'll be three at the end of October."

To the question, asked perhaps with a gesture toward her belly, "And when will this one arrive?" she would have said, "Beginning of October."

"Well, I guess you're keeping busy."

She must have laughed and said, "Yes, and there are three others. The oldest will be six at the end of November." Four children, five and under; one more on the way. My sisters and brother and I arrived, if not quite like clockwork, close to it. A gap of seventeen, eighteen, nineteen months separates each of us from the next. My mother planned on having seven children.

Everything had happened so fast. In 1944, just ten years earlier, the war was still going on. My mother was a junior at Radcliffe, walking across the Yard with a green book bag containing her copies of *The Canterbury Tales* and Pound's *Cantos* slung over her shoulder, "Mary Donovan, Bertram Hall" written on the flyleaves in blue-black fountain pen ink. Nearly every morning, through the open window of her dorm room, the words, "The uniform of the day will be the regular uniform of the day," drifted in from the PA system set up in the Yard, telling the students in ROTC what to wear. It was a phrase she would sometimes repeat to us when it was time for us to get out of our pajamas and into our clothes or out of our clothes and into our pajamas.

In April of 1945, on the radio, somber music played. "This morning, at 5:37 A.M., President Roosevelt died suddenly at Warm Springs. . . ." Truman was inaugurated with all the pomp of a shotgun wedding. A few months later the music was rousing. Germany had surrendered. And then the atom bombs were dropped on Japan. All through the fifties, on every calendar, May 8 had "V E Day" printed on it in red letters and August 14, "V J Day": victory in Europe, victory in Japan.

My father came home from the Pacific, met my mother but then could not find her again, because Bertram Hall had been shut down when the roof fell in. They ran into each other on the street in Cambridge. My mother graduated from Radcliffe, got a job at Harvard University Press, shared a flat on Beacon Hill with two other girls. Meat was still hard to get, she would tell us later. "What did you eat for dinner?"—dinner without meat being an unimaginable concept. "Sometimes we had peanut butter," she'd say, and I'd imagine peanut butter, formed into the shape of a roast and set on the pale blue glass platter on which our Sunday roasts were served, being carved into slices, a slice set on each plate. The three Boston career girls would have cut their slices of peanut butter with dinner knives and then lifted them to their lips with forks, interspersing bites of peanut butter with the boiled potatoes and boiled peas that surely must have accompanied the peanut butter roast.

In my fantasy they played the roles of women in 1940s movies. There would be the sharp-tongued older girl, all of twenty-six or twenty-seven, wise to the ways of the world; she'd of course be dark haired, blowing a stream of cigarette smoke out her nose. Another roommate played the ingenue, curly haired, dimpled, blond. Of course my mother must have been the lead, the girl torn between love and career. I will be able to imagine my mother's life so well because after I've had surgery I will lie in bed and watch old movies on TV: *His Girl Friday, Stage Door, I Was a Male War Bride, Adam's Rib.*

In December 1947, my mother and father were married at the Episcopal Church in Peterborough, New Hampshire, my mother in a long ivory gown, my father in a cutaway tux. For wedding presents they got Blue Willow china and silent butlers—flat-bottomed bowls in pewter and silver with lids, into which one could empty table crumbs and ashtrays. Everyone smoked then. Sandra was born in November 1948; Susan in May 1950; I was born in October 1951; Jane in March 1953. The years passed in a blur of diapers and nursing and Pablum and laughter and fatigue.

They moved from Cambridge, Massachusetts, to Alton, New Hampshire, where I was born, to upstate New York; my father went from being a graduate student to a school principal to an assistant professor; another war began, this time in Korea.

A few months before those late August, early September, days of 1954, we had moved out of "the units," former army barracks that had been moved to an open field on the north side of Hamilton. The postwar housing shortage was still going on, and Colgate's young faculty families took up residence in these square white clapboard buildings with their thin high windows and thin walls. We children played in the scrub yards where our mothers hung wash—sheets and cloth diapers and dishcloths along with our playclothes and occasional stiff-skirted party dresses—to dry on lines strung between rough, teetering wooden poles. My mother quoted Shakespeare around the house: About to clean the bathroom, she'd say, "Once more into the breach, dear friends." Gathering us together for a trip to the Grand Union—we waited in the car while she shopped—she'd say, "We few, we happy few, we band of brothers."

To this day I need only say, "the units," and my mother will sigh deeply and say, because she is so determinedly upbeat, "I was so happy to leave there."

By the late summer of 1954, we had moved into that farmhouse with slate gray–green shingles outside Hamilton. Winter days so cold the station wagon wouldn't start, my father would walk to the college on the other side of town with our dog, Poly, trotting after him. (No, we'd later have to explain to people. He wasn't named Poly because I'd had polio. He was named after the title character in *The Roly-Poly Puppy*.)

Six maple trees demarcated the front lawn of our new home. Behind the house was a long ridge, with a rutted dirt path leading out to an elm that stood alone just below its crest, looking like a ballerina with her arms raised in a circle above her head. Off the dirt path was a rusted piece of farm equipment, made to be pulled by horses, with a seat for the farmer and iron hooks behind for furrowing the soil. My mother would look at that piece of farm equipment and say, "Oh, if only we had found that during the war, when we were collecting scrap metal. We would have been so happy."

Those cycles of my childhood: a round of fall birthdays and a round of spring birthdays, my mother saying, "The uniform of the day will be the regular uniform of the day," and "We few, we happy few, we band of brothers," and "If only we'd found that when we were collecting scrap metal during the war."

The *New York Times* arrived at our house by mail a day late. In late August and early September 1954, the *Times* spoke of the Red regime in Peiping, as Beijing was then called, while the ads showed line drawings of women in impossibly steep heels and with equally impossible slim waists, petticoats with tiers of ruffles, a "ribbon" girdle in six delectable colors: lemon, lime, pink raspberry, pale blueberry, vanilla white, and licorice black. Children's summer camps would not be listed in the New York Commerce Department's directory unless a sworn affidavit was submitted as to their "non-subversive" nature. A Times Square raid had netted "rowdies, hoodlums, and undesirables." Noting that the price of coffee had risen sharply—a pound then cost between $1.18 and $1.42—an article titled "A Thriftier Cup of Coffee" recommended mixing coffee with such concoctions as chicory or Buisman's Famous Dutch Flavoring. A novel called *Chantal* was reviewed, translated from the French, the story of the title character, "originally a vain, unscrupulous ignorant young woman . . . reformed by her experience of illness and suffering." Sen. Joseph McCarthy was facing Senate censure for his conduct at the hearings investigating the army. President Eisenhower, in an obviously posed photograph, gazed at the bill he'd just signed, outlawing the Communist Party. An Alabama elementary school had barred twenty-three Negroes, paving the way for a court challenge to legal segregation.

And, on Friday, August 27, the *Times* noted that 2,207 cases of polio had been reported in the previous week, a rise of 15 percent from the previous week. The National Foundation was rushing respirators and iron lungs to hard-hit areas.

Summer was polio season. Air-conditioning was rare in those days. In the summer you were hot almost all the time, and by August nearly everyone had slipped into a state of languid torpor. Gaggles of folks sat on the porches of white clapboard houses, tenement stoops, country verandas. They ate summer fruit that the heat threatened to send from ripeness to decay in the space of an afternoon. Boys spat watermelon seeds at one another; flat-chested tomboys with dirty elbows sneaked off to swimming holes; kids danced in the jets from opened fire hydrants. Everything was sun drenched and freckle faced. Only the threats of polio and Communism lurked. Every summer the mothers told their children not to go swimming—they might get polio—not to drink from public water fountains, and if they couldn't wait until they got home, for heaven's sake, not to sit down on the seats of public toilets. The fathers told them never to sign a petition, your name might end up on some Communist list, especially not if the petition used words like "freedom" or "justice" or "free speech." Watch out. Give to the March of Dimes, wash your hands with good, strong soap, and never sign anything except a loyalty oath.

Who is she, this girl who will be three in October, whom I can track only with suppositions, *I must have seen . . . My mother must have said . . .* extrapolating backward from later memories?

When I was in my forties I received a writing fellowship and got to live in an ugly prefab 1950s cabin in one of the most beautiful places on earth, the mountaintop ranch where D. H. Lawrence lived outside Taos, New Mexico. Every morning I made a cup of strong, strong coffee and doused it with sugar and half-and-half because I hate the taste of coffee and drink it only for its drug effect, and walked out onto the deck. I looked down at the scrubby yard in front of me, the split-rail fence marking the field where Sassafras and Ebony, the caretaker's two horses, munched grass and flicked their tails lazily at flies. My friend Jeff, who later died of AIDS, talked about coming to visit me there but ended up not making the trip. When I was anticipating his arrival, I imagined him standing there on the porch next to me while I drank my coffee. We would have watched the horses ruminating in the field beyond the yard, seen the wild iris, and heard the shrill chirps and clicks of insects. Later, after he'd died, I supposed that when I was eighty I'd have forgotten that he never actually made it. The fantasy would grow seamlessly into memory, and it would be no different than if he had come and stood next to me there, smelling the earth, looking out at Sassafras and Ebony and the wild irises.

Every morning on the porch I looked up at a mountain in the distance, which appeared to be a color that occupied some equidistant space between purple and green and gray and imagined that on that opposite mountain, a woman stared at my mountain, which to her appeared as a clear, uncluttered form, a color equally distant from gray and green and purple. Maybe she stood on the deck of a 1950s prefab like me; maybe she was ecologically conscious and had built her house out of old tires or bales of hay. Were there trees on her mountain? Or maybe it was drier there, with a few stubborn, scrubby pines clinging to rock?

That past is like the mountain: hazy, beautiful, almost an illusion. Who is that girl with my name, my birth date, my genes, my first (almost) three years of history; the girl with my mother and my father and my sisters, my brother tucked inside my mother? Who is that girl who in late August and early September 1954 must have stood on the front porch of our house in Hamilton and looked past the six maples in the yard, past the line of weeping willows, at the house in the distance, which had once been red but was now faded to gray mottled with red? Did she stick her nose in one of the Blue Willow coffee cups with a half inch of cold black coffee in the bottom that my mother left here and there around the house? Did she take an experimental sip, then spit out the bitter liquid? Did she see the Indian paintbrushes, rust red and bright yellow, alongside the road? When, in late August, her parents took her out on a sailboat on Saranac Lake, did the feel of the wind on her face scare her, or did she laugh with a toddler's delight in the new? Did she believe her mother when she told her that everyone used to be a baby—not just her mother and father but even her grandmother and grandfather? Did she really believe that her mother was growing a new baby inside of her?

Years later, nine months pregnant, dreaming every night of schools of fish and stately vast houses, I will smell a rich fecund smell coming from between my legs, a smell my body has never given off before, yet familiar. Did I smell that smell when my mother stopped in at Streeter's to buy a spool of thread or a darning egg, and I pressed my face against her leg, clutching at her skirt, nose close to her crotch, while someone cooed, "What pretty blue eyes! How old is she?" and my mother answered, "She'll be three at the end of October." "And when's the next one due?"

My brother will be born at the beginning of October; I will turn three at the end of October.

But everything is about to change.

PREHISTORY

There is my personal prehistory, and then there is the disease's prehistory. For millennia polio remained one of humanity's nameless afflictions.

An ancient Egyptian stele sits inside a hermetically sealed glass case within a baroque edifice of a museum in Copenhagen, Denmark, thousands of miles from where it was carved three and a half millennia ago. The word *stele* is from the Greek, meaning "pillar" or "shaft." Adopted whole cloth into English: a word designed to conceal. The *stele* is oblong with a rounded top—the shape of a tombstone. For that is what it is, or was, before it became an artifact—the marker of Ruma's burial place, now housed in a Danish museum.

Etched into the stone, in stylized profile, is the figure of Ruma, a Syrian priest, leaning on a crutch, with an atrophied right leg and foreshortened foot. To his right are Ama, his wife, and their son, Ptah-m-heb. Worn hieroglyphics tell their names and the story of how Ruma was saved from death by the intercession of a goddess during his bout with the fever that left him with a paralyzed leg. This is almost certainly the first recorded case of the disease we now know as polio.

From the wall of New York's Metropolitan Museum, a barefoot boy smiles down on the visitors who shuffle beneath him. Jusepe de Ribera's seventeenth-century painting "The Beggar" shows a boy whose smile is simultaneously coy and enticing: *You think you are the one who is using* me—as an object of pity, as a means of feeling beneficent. Are you so sure about that? Perhaps I am the one who is taking advantage of you. His feet are bare—perhaps because he is poor, but also because he must display what he is offering to the gaze—of those from whom he once implored alms, of the painter, of the museum visitors—his oddly shaped foot, perhaps the result of polio. As I roll beneath him in my power chair, long flowing pants hiding the scars that are the result of surgery, the shape of my left leg, also distorted by surgery, I am once again in the position in which I find myself with disabled beggars. I conceal what they must show off.

In the market at Chichicastenango in Guatemala, I slip coins to a man who has an orthopedic brace like mine, only his is worn on the outside of his pants, while I hide mine. Outside a mosque in Tiranë, Albania, I bend over to pass folded *leks* to a woman who is an amputee, her skirt pulled up to reveal her stump.

In the early 1770s Sir Walter Scott—not then a "Sir," not then the author of *Ivanhoe* and the progenitor of the historical novel, just the toddler son of a middle-class Scottish family—had a nameless disease. He was struck with a fever. On the fourth day of that fever, his right leg was discovered to have "lost [its] power," which it was never to regain, his leg remaining "shrunk and contracted." "The impatience of a child soon inclined me to struggle with my infirmity, and I began by degrees to stand, walk, and to run." Had he lived in the city, Scott believed, he would have been "condemned to helpless and hopeless decrepitude," but the effect of country air and open space made him "a healthy, high-spirited, and, my lameness apart, a sturdy child."

In 1789 the disease gets a few-line mention in physician Michael Underwood's *A Treatise on the Diseases of Children; with General Directions for the Management of Infants from Birth* as "debility of lower extremities."

Scott also wrote of his childhood: "My father and mother had a very numerous family, no fewer, I believe, than twelve children, of whom many were highly promising, although only five survived very early youth."

Nothing so marks the gulf of separation between our age and that one just a few centuries before as the offhand way in which Scott dispenses with the deaths of seven siblings—more or less. Early deaths were part of the expected course of life. Those who survived the voyage from infancy to youth had almost invariably passed through bouts of fever and other afflictions. Polio, whether of the less common paralytic variety or presenting its more frequent face as an illness of fever and intestinal symptoms, would have been one of many of the undifferentiated diseases children endured. It must surely have killed some who got it, occasionally left others with some degree of paralysis, and passed almost unnoticed through others.

I DON'T REMEMBER

I don't remember waking up that morning in early September 1954. When I woke up that morning did my legs hurt? Did I call for my mother? Did she come into my room, crouch down next to my bed, ask me, "How do they hurt?" Did I say, "They tickle"? Did she say, "You probably just slept on them funny, sweetheart; that happens sometimes"? Did the thought of polio cross her mind? Or not—after all, there was no epidemic, Labor Day had just passed, the end of summer was the end of polio season.

I try to get back there by remembering the rooms of our farmhouse in upstate New York, but my father added onto the house while we lived there: What had been a bedroom became a TV room; another bedroom became part of the living room, a wall knocked down, so the physical setting, the anchor of memory, is jumbled.

All right, the kitchen then, that one room unchanged.

I don't remember, but Jane must have sat in the high chair with a pablum-splattered face and dirty bib: Everything must have been frosted with a layer of drool and grubbiness. There's my mother, maybe slicing open a package of bacon with a plastic-handled knife, peeling off the three strips of bacon my father has for breakfast every morning (bacon is expensive, so it's just for Daddy; on Sundays we are each allowed a single strip for breakfast), the bacon fat silky underneath her fingers. My mother lays the three strips in the skillet, turns on the burner of the electric stove while a child—maybe me?—pleads, "Pick me up, Mommy. Pick me up."

"Not now," she says, taking a sip of black coffee from her Blue Willow cup. She had started drinking coffee during the war, when everything was rationed, so she drinks it the way she got used to it: black. While my father, exactly five years and one day older than she, drinks it with top milk and sugar. Top milk is what floats on top of the glass bottles of non-homogenized milk the milkman delivers to our door several times a week. My mother pours it off into a cut-glass pitcher for my father to have in his coffee, and mixes the real milk in a one-to-one ratio with the Starlac powdered milk she buys at the Grand Union for the rest of us. Later on some 1950s development in food technology will cause these dried concoctions—dried milk, instant coffee, Kool-Aid—to dissolve more easily in water, and their packages will trumpet: *New! Crystallized! Freeze Dried! Dissolves Like Magic!* Back then she had to stir and stir and stir, and even after all that stirring, there was sometimes a chalky lump of Starlac in the milk that would catch in my throat and make me gag and wail.

What did I have for breakfast that morning? Maybe Rice Krispies—later that was my favorite breakfast. I liked to lean my ear down toward the bowl after my mother had poured in the milk and listen for the snap-crackle-pop the advertisements promised. Maybe I drank orange juice, too, the Grand Union brand my mother mixed up from the glop of frozen concentrate in a can. Maybe Jane is crying because she needs her diaper changed; maybe my mother is calling up the stairs to my father, "Jack! Jack! It's eight o'clock!" She turns down the burner under the bacon, warns me or Susan or Sandra, "Use both hands," or "Leave your sister alone," or "Move your juice back from the edge of the table."

She was always telling us to move things back from the edge of the table and to watch out for our hands when we shut the car door. Beware! Beware! Everything teeters on the brink of disaster. The thousand daily catastrophes of childhood: skinned knees, whacked funny bones, stubbed toes, quarrels, nightmares.

Maybe my mother said to Sandra, at five-almost-six the proud oldest, "Pour a glass of juice for your father and then put the pitcher back in the icebox." People still said "icebox," even though everyone had a refrigerator.

Later on real iceboxes—the sort that had once stood in my grandmother's kitchen, with their exteriors of polished mahogany or maple, patinated with thousands upon thousands of handprints, no longer redolent of the daily task of emptying the drip tray at the bottom, the wait for the iceman in the sultry July heat when the block of ice had long since melted away—will show up in antique stores, having crossed the line from seeming dowdy and slightly embarrassing to quaint, but then they were just memorialized in this lag of language.

"Both hands," my mother warns my sister Sandra as she lifts the pewter pitcher—a wedding present—from the metal table with its mottled gray Formica top. Perhaps, on the ridge of the hill above our house, a beetle carrying the fungus *Ceratocystis ulmi* has already laid her eggs in a gap between the bark and the wood of the elm tree, our eternally patient ballerina. Perhaps fungal spores are already adhering to the millions of bodies hatched from those eggs. The spores may be traveling into the xylem, the water-conducting veins of the tree, where, with yeastlike budding, they will reproduce, choking off the tree's lifeblood, causing its leaves to wilt and drop, its branches to die. Hordes of beetles will colonize the weakened tree, laying their eggs, which will, when hatched, carry more and more of *Ceratocystis ulmi* into the xylem, choking it further.

All that is not just invisible to us that Tuesday morning of September 7, 1954, but unimaginable—we have not yet heard of Dutch elm disease. Also unthinkable is the rapid replication taking place within my body. The virus that entered me some days or even weeks ago, worming its way into the very structure of one of my cells—in all probability one in my gut mucosa, from where, after wild replication, it had burst forth, shooting out, like a shower of sparks from an exploding firecracker, other viral particles, which in turn enter into other cells, repeating the process; spreading from there to the gray matter of my spinal cord, a rate of growth that makes geometric increase seem glacial. A single polio virus can enter a cell and hijack it, so it no longer functions as it once did but instead becomes a factory for reproducing the polio virus. In just one cell more than one hundred thousand copies of the virus have been produced. In my brain, in my gut, in my spinal cord, millions, tens of millions, hundreds of millions of cells have died, are dying, will die.

Of course such numbers are meaningless to me. Not yet three, how high could I count? Perhaps one, two, three, holding up a finger for each? As for the notion that my body should be an inviolable fortress, that this shroud of skin should mark off a self separate and distinct? After living forever in a world in which the words "my" and "her" did not exist—"my mouth," "her breast," "her arms," "my body"—I was still learning the first lesson that there was a "my" and a "her," that her will and my will were entirely separate things. And I was learning it with a vengeance. My most common words must have been "No," "Mine," and again, "No."

Did I say, "Susan touched my bowl. I don't want her touching that"? Did my mother respond with a general warning, "Everyone keep their hands to themselves," or "No squabbling"? Did I say, "Sandra's tickling me. Stop or I'll upchuck"? Did my brother, growing so big that he can scarcely move inside his amniotic cocoon, jostle my mother from within with an elbow or a knee?

Did I chorus, "Mommy, I don't feel well," continuing to spoon cereal into my mouth? Did my mother come over to me, lay a cool hand on my warm forehead, say, "You do feel a little warm, honey. Go lie down after you finish breakfast"? Or did she mean to come over and lay her hand on my head, but then get distracted—the bacon about to burn, the water the eggs were poaching in boiling over, my father entering the kitchen in his blue cotton pajamas?

A glass of orange juice, set too close to the edge of the table, might get bumped by an elbow and fall to the floor, shattering on the speckled linoleum floor with its bright spatter pattern, a design that prefigures Jackson Pollock's paintings. A bumblebee might make its way through a tear in the screen door and zip about our heads, causing us to flail our arms and holler. Our cat, Pinky, might leave a half-dead sparrow as an offering on the porch. These quotidian threatened disasters, even should they come to pass, are minor. Not like the decades before. No hungry tramps knock at back doors; no friends die on foreign shores. In this new world there is not just a chicken in every pot but a car in every garage—even if the cars here in Hamilton are not the ones associated with the fifties—no neon-colored cars—baby blue, tangerine, candy-apple red; no Cadillacs with enormous fins, two-tone Impalas. Folks here are solid. They remember the Depression all too well, so the cars are four or five years old, Pontiacs, Hudsons, painted in sedate dark blues and greens and blacks, still with the plump and stately postwar styling of the mid-forties, when the auto industry resumed civilian production. The bodies of these autos resemble those of the ample widows who bring tuna noodle casserole and rhubarb pies to the covered-dish suppers at the local Presbyterian church.

And then there's a fragment of narrative. Do I actually remember this, or is it just family lore I've heard repeated so often that it's become memory? I was playing house with my two older sisters—Sandra, the oldest, nabbed the part of the dad, and Susan would have been the mom, while I would have been willing to be the child, just for the glory of playing with them. Or maybe Gink, the life-size rag doll from the Sears Roebuck catalog was going to get to be the child, while I was being consigned to the role of baby. Where was Jane, the real baby of the family? A late walker, had she just started to take her first steps? Or was she still crawling around the house, working grit into the knees of her rompers? Maybe she was lying in her crib, crying so softly that my mother didn't hear her. To this day she has scars on her knees from rubbing her knees back and forth against her crib sheets as she wept almost silently, chafing her knees until they bled.

Before we could play house, a house had to be built, out of the orange-and-yellow cardboard building blocks called blockbusters that had also come from the Sears Roebuck catalog, and I had been ordered to wait in the bedroom until the house was built. Did I go there to and wait and wait and wait—wait for longer than it seemed possible to wait? (Throughout the years we lived in Hamilton, we went out to eat only once a year, when Grandma and Grandpa Finger came to visit, at Quack's Diner—"Going East / Going West / Quack's is the Best"—and I was amazed at the ability of the grown-ups to wait so patiently for their food. I could imagine myself when I was grown-up as a trapeze artist or a pilot, like Sky King, or a cowboy—but I could never imagine that I would be able to *wait* the way my parents could.)

Finally, when I couldn't stand it anymore, I must have walked into the room where they were playing and refused to budge. Susan took my arms and Sandra my legs, and they carried me back into the bedroom. Was I already wailing, "Mommy, Mommy, they won't let me play," when I fell down in the dining room and couldn't get up? Did my mother think I was having a temper tantrum and ignore me? How long did I lie there, my legs crumpled beneath me, before my mother realized that this was something more than toddler histrionics?

MYTHS OF ORIGIN

I

Where did it come from?

Where does the story begin?

Our family lore has it that my mother and oldest sister had polio first—the nonparalytic variety—because they had a stomach bug a few days before I came down with polio.

There we have it then: a place of beginning, an origin. I caught it from my mother or my sister. But like all origin stories (God made the world; the First People climbed up out of the Great Kiva; the Big Bang) it begs the question: And before that, what? Where had my mother and sister gotten it?

II

Tracing the origin to somewhere else is an almost inevitable move in the story of an epidemic. Where did it come from? Not here. In Daniel DeFoe's *Journal of the Plague Year,* he opens by saying that in September 1664 the plague was virulent in Holland. It had come there from Italy or the Levant, perhaps in goods from Turkey. In the United States, the beginning of AIDS is traced to Africa. In Africa, some claim that AIDS may have come from the West—perhaps through field trials of an experimental vaccine in the mid-1950s.

There. Not here.

III

Early summer in New York City. 1916. Lower Manhattan or Brooklyn.

The streets—many still unpaved—were crowded with barrows. Street stalls held bushel baskets and slit-open burlap sacks filled with beans—navy and cannellini and pinto and black—cornmeal, flour. Another one nearby offered used goods—darned socks, battered pans, scissors, ribbons, an empty picture frame or two, half-used spools of thread, books, what-have-you. A fruit seller displayed only apples and plums—not the plethora of choices that refrigeration and modern transportation have brought us. The smell of squid, eels, clams, and cod wafted out of a narrow storefront.

A chart showing the reported cases of infantile paralysis in New York lurches slowly upward throughout the month of June 1916. By July the number of new cases per day has reached fifty. That seems to have been the tipping point. The disease passes with stunning rapidity from the stage at which it had been largely a concern of public health officers and those directly affected by it into general awareness, and from general awareness into a cause of concern, and from there to outright panic.

News of the disease moved onto the front pages of the newspapers:

Bar All Children from the Movies in Paralysis War
25 More Deaths from Paralysis—Exodus of 50,000 Children
95 New Victims Here, 18 Deaths; Infant Scourge Covers 18 States

Suddenly evidence of the disease was everywhere. Houses and tenements where the disease had occurred were placarded with yellow-and-black quarantine signs. Even those who could not read, or could not read English, surely knew what the signs affixed to doorways meant. Thousands of pet cats were turned out by their owners after a rumor had gone around that they were carriers of the disease. They yowled at familiar doorsteps, demanding to be let back in, or prowled the streets, searching for food. Train stations were mobbed, as those who could—largely the wealthy and the middle class—sought to escape with their children from the city. Many made their escape only to find themselves turned back from outlying areas where they sought refuge by guards posted on highways and ports to keep outsiders from the town. In Hoboken, New Jersey, "Policemen were stationed at every entrance to the city—tube, train, ferry, road and cowpath—with instructions to turn back every van, car, cart, and person laden with furniture."

On July 18 the *Times* reported that "from noon Saturday until noon yesterday 150 families who attempted to enter Hastings-on-Hudson by train and automobile from New York were turned back by policemen stationed at every entrance to the village." New Yorkers leaving the city were spoken of as "refugees" and "fugitives." As far away as Mexico, travelers from New York found themselves quarantined.

A newspaper cartoon from that summer is captioned "A Scene in Any Suburb." Above it we see a girl labeled "New York Child" who, with her smock and beribboned hat, looks like a slightly older version of Madeline. She stands on a tree-lined street while locals—including mothers clutching their own children—run pell-mell from her, shooting looks back at her that combine fear and rage. The only figure coming toward her is a policeman, his truncheon raised above his head.

"No doubt many scenes which occurred in London during the great plague of 1665 were reenacted in our Long Island and Westchester towns," wrote one contemporary:

Deputy sheriffs, hastily appointed and armed with shot-guns, patrolled the roads leading in and out of towns, grimly turning back all vehicles in which were found children under sixteen year [*sic*] of age. Railways refused tickets to these selected youngsters, the innocent victims of ignorance and despair. Indeed, the notion was firmly held that below the magic age, called sweet at other times, there lurked the dread disease, whereas above it no menace existed for either the individual or the community.

In Middletown, New York, special prayers were offered in churches for paralysis patients—although all children under sixteen were excluded from the services.

In New York City, during the 1916 epidemic, the faraway place from which the disease had come was Italy. Never mind that the Ellis Island Quarantine Station stated that "no cases had been noticed among immigrants," and that there was "no record of epidemics in any of the towns of Italy." To those who called themselves native Americans, by which they meant those of good Northern European stock, the miserable, squalid apartments in which the Italian immigrants lived must have seemed hives of sickness, in which any number of diseases were stewed into virulence. And then there was the peasant habit—continued in New York—of not segregating animal and human life. Birds, goats, chickens, and pigs were kept in or near their tenement apartments. Sometimes whole tenement floors were given over to monkeys, which were rented to organ grinders. Imagine walking along the Bowery and hearing, issuing forth from within the dark walls of tenements, the screeching of monkeys, the snuffling of pigs, a rooster's triumphant call.

Soon the connection of "the infantile"—as it was sometimes called—with Italians was to become so firmly entrenched that the presence of an Italian with a portable merry-go-round "suspected of coming from an infected neighborhood" was enough to result in the police ordering the man—who was referred to only as "the Italian"—off the streets.

IV

But was that epidemic the origin of polio epidemics in the United States? No, before New York, there was an epidemic in Vermont in 1910. And before that, also in Vermont, an epidemic in 1894.

In the summer of 1894 the Otter Creek, which gives its name to the valley it runs through in Rutland County, Vermont, seemed to be moving at a particularly slow pace. Normally its waters, fed from the nearby Green Mountain range, were languid—but during that summer, a summer that would be remembered for an altogether different reason, the river was especially sluggish.

Could there be any connection between the pace of the river's waters and the strange disease that had appeared that summer? Like other epidemic diseases—cholera or typhoid or diphtheria—this one sometimes killed, sometimes did not. What was different about this disease was that when the acute phase of the illness had passed, many were left paralyzed. Even more puzzling was the fact that after a period of weeks or months the paralysis vanished in some. In others it did not.

A three-year-old boy had a fever lasting two or three days. When the fever ended he could not use his legs. Within ten days he could walk by holding on to a chair, and in three weeks' time he had fully recovered. Another three-year-old boy had a fever that followed a similar course: It lasted for a few days, and when it passed, he was left without the ability to walk. Although he regained function in his right leg, the other remained affected. Another child with a similar fever died on the sixth day.

What was most perplexing about this new spate of paralyzed children—and even some adults—was that, whatever was causing the paralysis, it did not seem to be a contagious disease. If it had been, it would have followed the expected pattern. One member of a family would have come down with a fever, with the additional symptoms of weakness and malaise and then paralysis, followed by the rest of the family in rapid succession. Perhaps one or two household members would escape the pestilence—those who, for some unknown reason, were immune. Instead, as Dr. Charles Caverly, a practicing physician in Rutland and the president of the Vermont State Board of Health, noted, "it has affected most invariably but a single member of a household." Certainly other people in the household may have been sick—a touch of diarrhea, perhaps some vomiting and stomach cramps, a slight fever—but in that age before refrigeration, such illnesses, especially in the summer months, attracted scant attention.

And then? Summer ended. As August turned to September and the daisies and red clover of summer gave way to the goldenrod and gentians of early autumn, the number of new cases lessened. By the time October came and the hillsides covered with maples and elms and oaks were in full color, the mysterious passage of this new paralysis through the towns had waned and then disappeared.

Caverly—one of a new breed of medical men who saw themselves as scientists and had set out to apply rigorous methods to the previously rough-and-tumble, seat-of-the-pants practice of medicine—set out to track down the root of this strange plague. He gathered facts, looked for a pattern. He tabulated nationalities; the age of the houses in which the paralyzed lived; whether those infected lived in a "detached house" or a "tenement house"; whether they kept dogs, cats, horses, cows, pigs, and hens; the proximity of animal quarters to the house; whether water was supplied by a well, a private aqueduct, or from the public supply; the families' sewer facilities—"dry closet" (outhouse) or connection to the public sewer. The family's medical history was collected and ranked; as were the occupations of the wage earner: "Blacksmith, Clerk, Engineer, Farmer, Fireman, Granite Cutter, Insurance, Iron Worker, Junk Dealer." No matter how hard Caverly looked, he couldn't find any pattern that led him closer to the cause of this baffling illness.

What Caverly did not realize was that the disease most often occurred in a nonparalytic form, as a brief intestinal disorder, and thus was spread by those who did not themselves give any sign of illness.

The time when Caverly was entering medicine was one of enormous optimism. In the past, miasmas had been seen as the cause of infectious diseases. Derived from a Greek word meaning "pollution and defilement," "miasma" refers to heavy, vaporous air. In the late 1870s the causative role of microbes in disease had been advanced—notably by Robert Koch and Louis Pasteur. Koch's postulates were elegant in their simplicity. A specific microorganism is always associated with a given infectious disease; the microorganism can be taken from the body of an infected animal and grown in the laboratory; it will subsequently cause the same disease in another animal. Infectious diseases no longer seemed diffuse and perplexing; they became not only comprehensible but preventable through social and medical interventions, notably vaccination. In this new conception disease was losing its moral and spiritual valence. This new way of conceptualizing illness was slowly overturning the older notion of filth as a cause of disease.

The golden disease-free future, which lay just beyond the horizon, would come about not only through medical progress but through broader social reforms.

When progress seemed so close at hand, how could this new disease be emerging? What was the cause of this epidemic? What had been its origin—and, just as important from an epidemiological perspective, why had it ended? How did it spread? Would a carrier like Typhoid Mary be found? Was it caused by some environmental exposure?

V

Stockholm, 1881. Lovely Stockholm, built on fourteen ribbons of island flung across a lagoon, the Venice of the North. The Swedes prided themselves on their progressive approach to health and social welfare. At first the epidemic seemed an aberration, a blip on the steady ascent into the paradise they were making here on earth. And for a few years it seemed that they were right: The strange new epidemic departed as mysteriously as it arrived.

And then, in 1887, it returned, more furiously than before.

And then it disappeared again.

In 1905 it came back. And then again in 1911.

In the United States polio was known as the "summer plague," but in Sweden it was called *höstens spöke,* "autumn's ghost."

Every time it seems we've come to the first epidemic, an earlier one is uncovered. In 1841 a physician visited the parish of West Feliciana in Louisiana and heard of a handful of children who had come down with a sudden paralysis:

> Whilst on a visit . . . my attention was called to a child about a year old, then slowly recovering from an attack of hemiplegia. The parents (who were people of intelligence and unquestionable veracity) told me that eight or ten other cases of either hemiplegia or paraplegia had occurred during the preceding three or four months within a few miles of their residence, all of which had either completely recovered, or were decidedly improving. The little sufferers were invariably under two years of age.

And before that: Worksop, England, 1835, where four cases of suddenly induced paralysis appeared in children who were treated by a Dr J. Badham, who reported on them in great detail in a contemporary medical journal. It may well be that there were more children who did not receive any medical care.

And before that: A Danish archaeological expedition in South Greenland excavated a cemetery that had belonged to a medieval Norse colony, Herjolfsnes, dating from the beginning of the fifteenth century, and discovered that six out of the twenty-five individuals examined had had diseases involving physical deformities suggestive of polio, and leading to the conclusion that a polio epidemic may have swept through the colony. Some of the people in Hieronymus Bosch's *The Procession of Cripples,* painted in 1500, were probably polio survivors.

And the ancient Greek physician Hippocrates, in his *Of the Epidemics,* writes of the island of Thásos, where one winter, "paraplegia set in, and attacked many, and some died speedily; and otherwise the disease prevailed much in an epidemical form."

Jane Smith, in her *Patenting the Sun,* expresses the explanation that held sway for so long:

> Put simply, paralytic polio was an inadvertent by-product of modern sanitary conditions. When people were no longer in contact with the open sewers and privies that had once exposed them to the polio virus in early infancy, when paralysis rarely occurs, the disease changed from an endemic condition so mild that no one even knew it existed to a seemingly new epidemic threat of mysterious origins and terrifyingly unknown scope.

However, studies of disability in developing countries undermine this view. Polio has a high prevalence in rural Uganda and India, where sanitary conditions are primitive. Polio epidemics seem to have come into view because we were looking for them. Shortly before the start of the twentieth century, infant mortality began to fall, and medical attention began to be paid to childhood illnesses. As Cotton Mather put it, in the colonial period a dead child was "a sight no more surprising than a broken pitcher." The combination of expecting children to survive childhood, a mass media that could spread the word of an outbreak, and a medical system that was geared to surveillance of childhood illnesses "created" epidemic polio.

On the shores of Lake Atitlán, some young men ask me that old familiar question: "What happened?" *¿Que pasa?* gesturing toward my legs. "Polio," I say, but they don't know the word. They are a little bit drunk. One of them asks, *¿Pollo?* and mimics, with two of his fingers, a chicken running around, and the others start laughing. "No, polio," I repeat. *Poliomyelitis.* "It's a sickness," I say in Spanish, but they are baffled. I know *polio* is the word in Mexican Spanish, but perhaps there's a different one here in Guatemala?

Later, on one of the ferries across the lake, I overhear some North Americans talking, one saying, "What we saw in that village wasn't just malnutrition but pure caloric insufficiency." I realize they are medical workers and ask them if there is a different word in Guatemala for polio. One of them looks it up in a pocket medical dictionary they have and tells me, no, there's no other word. Polio is a disease in a sea of diseases in Guatemala, in a land where malnutrition is a step up from caloric insufficiency.

VI

I go back to Hamilton, driving in a rental car I've picked up outside New York City. A hokey song echoes through my head, "The Green, Green Grass of Home," a prisoner awaiting execution, imagining his return home. *The old town looks the same,* the voice embedded in my head croons as I drive along the Thruway, the cruise control set five miles above the speed limit, past the blasted bedrock that lines the highway. I've seen a picture of downtown Hamilton on the Colgate Web site, and it looks as if it's hardly changed at all: the solid buildings made of deep red stone facing the town green are all still there; the Colgate Inn still stands, forthright and proper, across from the town green. The movie theater, where we paid 35 cents on Saturday afternoon to see *Bambi* or *The Snow Queen,* is still there. And then I realize there will be ramps, curb cuts, handicapped parking spaces: the architecture of the town will recognize my existence.

"Exit in two miles," the synthesized female voice says from the GPS. "Exit highway in one mile."

There to meet me are my mama and papa. . . .

"Exit highway now."

And then I am in the landscape that was my first landscape: low and lush, vines wrapping themselves around telephone poles and guy wires and fence posts. Every fall each maple sends thousands of samaras, its seeds with two translucent, featherlike wings, helicoptering down toward the earth underneath. My best friend, Debby, and I used to sit under the trees, splitting the embryonic tree casings open with our short fingernails, examining the frail curled shoots. A brood of saplings surrounds each maple that lines the sides of the road. Ferns—looking remarkably similar to the plants they had evolved from, the first forms of plant life established on land—can be glimpsed in the darker loamy recesses. I've grown used to cloudless California skies, the clean, insistent sunshine. Here the sky is flecked with cirrus clouds, dappling the light.

I drive past farms named Sweet Meadow, Saddleback Ranch, Cherry Valley. A few still have circular stone barns, which once stored hops used in brewing beer. I drive past abandoned houses and farms, their weathered boards once painted barn red or whitewashed. Here, as across the country, individual farms are shutting down, their herds and lands being absorbed by agribusiness—but I don't want to romanticize those disappearing family farms. In the 1950s the farmers around us were still in their honeymoon period with the chemical companies that made pesticides and fungicides. DDT was—like the Salk vaccine—a miracle. When my mother assigned her students at Earlville High School, ten miles south of Hamilton, the sons and daughters of dairy and truck farmers, Rachel Carson's groundbreaking critique of pesticides, *Silent Spring,* they grumbled. Their fathers said she was worse than a Communist. And none of the vegetable growers could have survived without the underpaid labor of migrant farm workers, who rode into town on old yellow school buses, picked beans and strawberries, and headed south after the first frost. All the migrant workers who came to Hamilton were African American, and the shanties on the edge of town where they lived were little better than slave quarters. I remember the sense of shock I had when we drove past one of the camps at night, the migrant workers gathered around a campfire, laughing and singing. I knew that the way they were forced to live was wrong, and I dutifully felt sorry for them— and *oh!* my umbrage at their having so much fun. I had imagined that when they finished work, they sat glumly in their cabins, staring at the walls, and grieving over the injustices they were forced to endure.

The poorest farm kids also lived in squalid conditions. They might come to school with adhesive tape holding their shoes together or wearing the same dress day after day after day. Rumors went around school about the cruelties visited on some of these girls by their fathers—men who were humiliated by their utter lack of power beyond their few acres of mortgaged farmland and who paid back their humiliations at home. I remember in particular that one of my sister Susan's classmates had been forced by her father to drown the kittens the family cat had given birth to. She had sobbed about it on the bus the next day. Word of what had happened traveled around the school bus, and her father's action was universally condemned. After all, one of her brothers would have been happy to do it—or, I now realize, at least have pretended to be enjoying himself.

The remaining paint on these abandoned barns feathers into the grain of the wood; the metal roofs are rusting. I drive past yellow-and-black diamond-shaped signs showing leaping deer, cattle, a farmer driving a tractor. Tire swings hang from sturdy branches. Milk cans, which I remember being picked up by flatbed trucks from the ends of driveways every morning, have now become decorative: They serve as planters or, filled with cement, hold two-by-fours with a mailbox on top. Wild lilacs bloom in front of tarpaper shacks. A dead deer, its sack of guts hanging out of its belly, lies by the side of the road. I drive through the plainly named towns surrounding Hamilton: Pooleville, Hubbardsville, Earlville. Crooked Hill Road, Johnny Cake Hill Road, Hardscrabble Road. Stone fences, fields lying fallow, squares of alfalfa and clover; springtime fields with the first shoots pushing up through the furrowed ground. One deserted house I pass has a broken window through which protrude the slats of a tumbledown Venetian blind, which has torn through the screens. The tattered screens hang like Spanish moss. It could be a sculpture by Eva Hesse. Looking into the hayloft of an abandoned barn, I see piles of plastic detritus—green plastic trash bags, topped by a child's plastic tricycle.

I pull into the handicapped parking space behind the Colgate Inn as the voice from the rental car GPS tells me, "You have arrived."

I had called the Colgate Library to make sure they had copies of the *Mid-York Weekly* going back to the early 1950s. Yes, the voice on the other end of the telephone says. He also tells me that the library is in the midst of moving. I ask if they are still in the turreted building on the edge of campus, which I thought was the most beautiful building on earth—it reminded me of Sleeping Beauty's castle in the Disney cartoon.

No, it has been decades and decades since the library has been in that building. And then I remember that a new library was being built just as we were moving away in the early 1960s. Now the new library has become old, and they are moving out of that.

At the Colgate Library I park in the handicapped parking space by the accessible entrance. A gaggle of trucks and machinery outside the door, men in hard hats, plastic tarps, a sign reading: "Warning! Asbestos Removal in Progress!"

"Hi!" I call out. I'm warm and friendly wherever I go, meeting the gazes of strangers on the street—interrupting their looks before they can become stares—offering my cheery "Good Mornings!" and "Hellos!" A coping strategy so many of us develop. Think of the ebullient personality that was part of Roosevelt's response to his disability, the iconic image of him with his head tilted back, a cigarette holder between his teeth, grinning.

"I need to get into the library," I tell one of the construction workers.

"It's pretty hard to get through here."

"I'm not particularly wild about going where you're doing asbestos removal. . . . I can walk a little bit." I end up getting wheeled up the hill, climbing a few steps hanging on to the railing with both hands, while the man who has pushed me up the too-steep hill lifts my ultralight wheelchair up the steps. "Thank you so much," I say.

Some days my life feels like a series of *thank-yous*. *Thank you*, to strangers for holding doors open for me, to bus drivers for not driving past me at the bus stop, to those who get up from their seats on the bus so I can move into the wheelchair space. *Thank you so much. Thank you, I really appreciate your help*, to people who carry my chair up a few steps, tilt my chair back, and bump me up where there's no curb cut. I can say it in French: *Merci, merci beaucoup*; in Spanish, *Gracias, Usted es muy amable; Thank you, you are very kind*; in Italian, *Grazie, grazie, mille grazie. Thank you, thank you, a thousand thank-yous*. In Portuguese, *Obrigada*. For a while I could say it in Greek and in Albanian, but now I have forgotten.

Disability puts you on a different plane with everyday interactions. The photographer Dorothea Lange, most famous for her Depression-era images, especially the iconic migrant mother, was a survivor of polio who walked with a noticeable limp. She felt that her disability had been an enormous aid to her as a photographer: "When I was working . . . with people who were strangers to me, being disabled gave me an immense advantage. People are kinder to you." She may have pulled up at a migrant camp or sharecroppers' cabin in what to our eyes, glazed by abundance, may seem just an ordinary, serviceable car, but to them must have looked like a magnificent vehicle. When she clambered out of the car, her subjects saw her vulnerability. "It puts you on a different level than if you go into a situation whole and intact."

Sometimes I appreciate the way my disability knocks down the ordinary barriers, but sometimes I get tired of strangers feeling free to ask me personal questions or to tell me their own stories of hard luck and tribulation.

Once inside the library, I wheel my way past cardboard cartons, upturned maroon couches stacked against walls, making my way to the periodicals room, where I am handed the bound copies of the *Mid-York Weekly*, its logo the outline of the state with a flint-tipped arrow piercing it in the middle.

I turn the yellowed newsprint carefully, arriving at September 8, 1954, expecting to see news of my getting polio. After all, wasn't a single case enough to have put a community on alert, everyone holding his or her breath, waiting for the next child to fall ill? Wouldn't one anxious woman have called another, each holding the enormous receiver of a black telephone, *Have you heard?* I can imagine the women, having opened their screen doors, standing in doorways, aprons tied around the waists of their full-skirted dresses; the farm women perhaps wearing the cotton housedresses that were shown at the back of the women's clothing section in the Sears Roebuck catalog in black-and-white photographs; perhaps some of the faculty wives wearing dresses that had been bought on a yearly trip to Boston or New York City; all of them calling their children home. I can hear a canopy of words weaving itself across the air of the town: "Dilys!" "Tommy!" "Johnny!" "Cindy! "Pam!" "Hilary!" "Mary!" "Duncan!" "Laurie!" "Come home!" "Come home!" And then those women— whether farmwives, who'd heard the alarm clatter at four thirty in the morning and gone downstairs to start breakfast before waking everyone else up for their chores, or women who had slept in until seven—would gather their children close to them, sheltering them, warning them not to stray, to stay away from the movie theater and especially not to go out to the lake.

But there is no mention of this solitary case of polio. On the front page is a story about a visit from a lodge leader, shown in a photograph with a tasseled fez atop his head, the Grand Monarch of the Supreme Council, Mystic Order of Veiled Prophets of the Enchanted Realm, who gave a talk—complete with sound pictures—about the work being done by his organization for cerebral palsy. On the lower-right-hand corner of the front page, it notes that a migrant camp laborer has been sentenced to sixty days for assault on another migrant camp laborer. A few weeks later another migrant camp laborer will also be also sentenced to sixty days, in that case for stealing a sweatshirt valued at $1.39 from a local store.

At the state fair a Morrisville boy has won a prize for his Brown Swiss calf—bred on the Hi-Ho Farm—given by the State Holstein, Ayrshire, Guernsey, Jersey, Brown Swiss and Milking Shorthorn Association. The State Fair continues with prizes to be offered by the County Poultry Judging Team and in the Tractor Operating Contest. Inside is an advertisement for an "Orlon-Nylon Suit—weighs less than one pound. Wash it—dry it—wear it twenty minutes later!"

I keep paging through those copies of *Mid-York Weekly*, looking for a mention of me, my polio, but there is none. Covered-dish suppers are held at the Presbyterian church. Children are born—including, on October 12, a son to Mr. and Mrs. John Finger.

I leave the new library, rolling down the hill to where my car is parked. The new library has become old and out of date. The asbestos—once thought to be a lifesaver for its fire-retardant properties—turned out instead to be a bane, seeding deadly cancers.

VII

And the virus itself? Where did it come from?

First some words of definition. Since both bacteria and viruses are microscopic and cause disease, they are often assumed to be close relatives, an association made evident not just in common parlance, in which they are lumped together as "germs" and "bugs" but also in scientific language, in which they are spoken of as "microbes" and "pathogens."

Their fundamental nature is different, however. Bacteria are living organisms, while viruses—mere strands of RNA or DNA—exist on the boundary between the living and the nonliving. Although viruses reproduce themselves, they are not cells and are incapable of reproducing outside a living thing.

Bacteria were present in that teeming soup from which all life evolved, which makes them our venerable ancestors. Without bacterial decay—the decomposition of proteins—everything and everyone that had ever existed on earth would still be here. In a world without rot, everything stays. Every leaf that's ever fallen from a tree still exists, as does every McDonald's burger wrapper, every turd. An image flashes across my mind—the unrotted bodies of every single human being who has ever lived, stacked like cordwood, in sheds and mausoleums that stretch for miles and miles. Of course human life would never have been possible without that continual replenishment of the soil by bacterial decomposition. That life would be impossible without death is not a grand cosmological statement but a simple, microscopic one. Only occasionally are bacteria our antagonists, colonizers wreaking havoc where they colonize, creators of bronchitis, pneumonia, meningitis. Mostly, bacteria sustain our lives by being the Great Recycler.

But viruses? They sow not, neither do they reap. They are pure strands of DNA or RNA, wearing only a coating, called a capsid.

The polio virus is made up of RNA, the abbreviation for ribonucleic acid. "Ribonucleic acid." How that phrase seems to float above us in the stratosphere of what the dictionary describes as "International Scientific Vocabulary." I want to pull those words down closer, to crack them apart, to see where they come from, what's inside them. The "ribo" comes from the German word *die Ribose,* which refers to a white crystalline five-carbon sugar. The German language borrowed the word *Ribose* from the English "arabinose," meaning "Arab sugar." The sugar itself derived, as was the word, from "gum arabic." A substance, something you can see and touch, the gum given off by the type of acacia tree known as *Acacia senegal* to heal its bark after damage, forming a tear-shaped exudate. The word "nucleus," center, comes from a Latin word *nux,* nut, meaning "kernel," "inner part." The word "acid" is derived from the Latin word *acidus,* sour; the *ac-* root going back to the Greek for "sharp, pointed." We can break those remote words apart and find that at the core of them lie the names of things that can be touched, eaten; a sharp feeling in the mouth, a gummy substance from a tree, a pod cracked open to reveal the nut within.

There is another name for the poliomyelitis strand of ribonucleic acid: A name that begins UUAAAACAGCUCUGGGGUUGUACCCACCCC and goes on for another 6,940 letters, each letter indicating the presence of the proteins adenine, guanine, cytosine, or uracil. The virus's true name might be the babbling of a baby or a word from *Finnegans Wake*.

The virus itself, that pure stripling of genetic material, cared not one whit about the names hung on it. It merely entered the cells of my body, an unwelcome guest that, without hearing "Take off your coat and stay awhile," nonetheless did just that, sloughing off its coating of protein, revealing itself to be stark naked underneath; not just unclothed but barer than bare, without those weighty encumbrances of flesh and bone and slithery guts with which—depending upon your point of view—either we lug about our genomes or our genomes lug us about. Everything inessential had been stripped away, and there was just a pure genetic command.

Where did the virus come from originally? Scientists now believe that viruses are escaped fragments of nucleic acids that have assumed an independent existence. Perhaps they escaped from bacteria, or perhaps they escaped from our genome. A wayward sister who set out on her own, a prodigal son; offspring now returning. This may be why the virus knows us so well, why it fits so perfectly into the very marrow of our cells. Perhaps long ago it was part of us. Following the command of a god who has told it to be fruitful and multiply, it replicates, it replicates, replicates, replicates, replicates. It is what a virus does, the way dogs sniff, cows chew, humans think.

TELLING SYMPTOMS

What do I remember of my initial experience of polio?

A memory so vague as to be less than dreamlike. Eerie gowned figures. A glass wall.

After that, a single clear memory of the hospital in Syracuse, where I spent the acute phase of my illness. I was no longer in a solitary room but a ward that I shared with three or four other children. One of them, an older girl—four, or maybe even five, she seemed almost an adult to me—was displaying her toys, which she had stashed in a white pillowcase, to another child. As she pulled out a square jack-in-the-box, she said, "Don't let Anne see this or she'll start crying." I wanted to tell her that I am no longer scared of this jack-in-the-box, although the reason she had it is that I had wailed in terror when it was given to me and the lid of the box flew open and the clown lurched out at me.

And one more foggy memory: a green tiled room, to which I have been transferred because I am having an asthma attack.

Both of those are later, when the acute stage of the illness has receded.

Of the acute stage, when I was in the grip of the "common, acute viral disease," the "brief febrile illness," only a masked-and-gowned figure, a glass wall.

Of what happened to my body itself, of that I have no memories.

———

In the grip of polio fever, sportswriter Jim Marugg hallucinated that his body had been taken apart during the night, and he was unable to find its pieces. He called to his wife, " 'Sylvia! Syl! I can't find my body.' " He ran into the garage—maybe his body was in the old trunks or cartons out there. In the garage he jumped in the car and realized that he had his legs. Now for his hands. Maybe hiding the pieces of his body was a practical joke his coworkers were playing on him. Suddenly he was at the newsroom, but no one there seemed able to see him. He knew he had to find his body, show it to them, or else he would lose his job. In the elevator he pushed a button. All right, hands and legs! Okay, now all he needed was his body itself:

> I was somewhere trying to put all the pieces of my body together again. I'd lose a piece and chase after it . . . vexation, weariness, pain and horrible confusion. Over and over and over again the same routine. Finally triumph, or almost triumph—I had all the parts but my eyes. Now if I could just find them I could see to put myself together and be whole again.

Charles Mee was fourteen when he had polio: "As the neurons in my body died one by one during those two weeks, I felt relentless pain, like the pain of a tooth being drilled without Novocain, but all over my body."

And Lorenzo Milam, a one-man band of an author, who never met a metaphor he didn't like, evokes in *The Cripple Liberation Front Marching Band Blues,* the universe of fever, a hothouse where sensations blossom into hallucinations:

> My brain is a bird. A bird trapped in a pale cage, a cage of bone. The fires are raging all about, and the bird, in fear, escapes from the cage of bone . . . frantic, eyes shiny with fear, beak ajar, beats wings against the corners of the room. . . . The inferno consumes the body, lays waste to the cells, and, in the process, plumbs the deepest shadows of the mind. Seamless grounds open, vampires and grayish beasts come swarming forth, extricating themselves from the pits. Figures lurch out of caves hollowed in the ground. . . . Sticky feet beat small rhythms across the figure wrapped in white linen. From time to time, masks lean out of chambered porticoes, jaws open volcanoes to release clouds of words into a barren sky.

I do know that every now and again I have a fantasy in which everything humanity has come to rely on disappears. I don't mean things humanity has come to rely on like houses, cars, cell phones, highways, power wheelchairs, supermarkets. I mean everything we have come to rely on like gravity, one's sense of up and down, causality, time itself.

It is as if the sensation you have during the first fraction of a second at the beginning of an earthquake went on forever and ever. Or, walking down a flight of unfamiliar steps in the dark, taking a step down a stair that isn't there. That sensation. But not ending a fraction of a second later when your conscious mind kicks in: It's an earthquake. You've passed the last step. That feeling, going on and on forever, while you are hurtled through a wild and directionless landscape, and everything around is being hurtled too. The only thing I can hold onto are the words "What's happening?" Some great hand has pulled the plug on our cosmos, and we are being sucked away into an alternate universe. Since there is no time in this other universe, we are never quite there.

Is this a memory of polio?

In the fifties and early sixties it never occurred to anyone that the interiors of hospitals might be painted in bright primary colors. They were pale brown, unnatural green, like the walls of elementary schools. The nurses were, of course, dressed in white, and the doctors wore white coats over their dun brown or gray suits. At three o'clock each day, when my mother came, she brought with her not just her familiar smell but a splash of color.

The other day I bought daffodils and lemons at a produce market. When I glance over to my sideboard and see them there, the lemons in a glazed blue bowl from Mexico, the daffodils stuck in an old-fashioned milk bottle, I feel what Alan Greenspan would doubtless term irrational exuberance at the sight of them. When I was living in Detroit and having a bad day, I would wheel across the street to the Detroit Institute of Arts to stare at "my" van Gogh—the portrait of Postman Roulin—loving especially the brilliant blue of his cap and jacket.

Now that MRIs have brought the living brain into view, it is possible to slide people who have had polio into the enormous tubes of those machines and peer inside our brains.

The music piped over headphones cannot drown out the bonging made by this machine, only give the person being imaged another sound on which to concentrate. The only other time I have experienced a similar sound was while visiting a Welsh slate mill, preserved as it had been at the beginning of the Industrial Revolution. The machinery gave off a similar, insistent *thud-thud-thud*—and I thought that Blake's "dark Satanic mills" was not, after all, a bit of religious-romantic exaggeration but a clean and apt description.

We can be slid into those machines, and a computer-constructed picture of our postpolio brains is generated, sometimes rendered in shades of gray but sometimes jazzed up with Day-Glo colors, fluorescent yellows, electric blues.

When I lived in England, I used to see the brains of cows and pigs set out for sale behind the glass of the butcher's case. Headcheese, sweetbreads. This was back in the days before offal became hip, when it was just food for those who couldn't afford real meat. A white cow's brain is not so different from my brain. Neurological tissue, wrinkled from being crammed into the shell of my skull, like clothes stuffed into a suitcase.

Those MRIs reveal encephaliticlike lesions peppering the brains of those of us who had polio, with an affinity being shown for the *substantia alba,* or white matter, rather than the *substantia grisea,* or gray matter, leaving our higher-level cognitive functioning intact. A medical journal article I read about this contends that the main site of infection in acute polio was the brain and that the nerves of the spinal column were affected as an "afterthought." I read these words and allowed myself to be amused at the notion of viral consciousness, but for the next few days I found myself touching my head and thinking—wormwood, Swiss cheese.

During the initial bout with polio, I must have been in the grip not only of unremembered pain and unremembered fever but of some wild forces at work deep in my brain.

For a while, when I was a kid, I wanted to be an archaeologist. I read about carbon dating, Heinrich Schliemann's excavations of Troy, how archaeologists worked with patient slowness. Although what they did in the field was called a dig, they didn't thrust shovels into the earth, but instead, working meticulously with fine-toothed brushes, cleared away accumulations of dust and dirt, taking note not just of the uncovered shards and fragments themselves but of the way each one lay in relation to another. I was fascinated by the past, by things that were buried, meanings that could be known only by a process of slow and patient decryption.

For Christmas one year my mother gave me *Voices in Stone,* about the deciphering of ancient languages, the text itself translated from the German and thick with Germanic romanticism. It began with talk of "the Word, the divine spark of coherent speech . . ." There was more about wresting from the Sphinx the key to her riddles, and those who deciphered languages were said to have "broken" them. I loved words I didn't understand, loved them for their mystery, their possibilities: "mnemonic . . . quipus . . . ideographic . . . philology . . . hieratic . . . syllabary . . . calamus . . . lucubrations . . . Monophysitism . . . obelisks . . . perspicacity." I loved to leaf through the book and see the line drawings that showed how Sumerian pictograms had evolved in cuneiform, or to stare at the Egyptian hieroglyphics, with their stylized legs and eyes, the representations of scarabs and vipers and cobras, of vultures, quail, chicks, owls, and falcons.

I wanted to be the one to break the languages that were still unknown—the symbols of Easter Island, runes etched on a few wooden tablets; the tongue of the Etruscans.

Was my desire to know what had been erased from memory, to read forgotten languages, another telltale symptom?

In the face of bureaucratic ineptness, I often experience not just the expected annoyance but utter despair. Waiting on hold with the Department of Motor Vehicles is not anyone's idea of fun, but I can feel bereft in that situation, utterly powerless, and an impotent rage flows from that sense of powerlessness. I will never get through, I will spend the rest of my life with this telephone receiver pressed to my ear. Is that an echo of the despair and rage I experienced in the hospital, at the numbing routines that surrounded me?

I am acutely aware of the strength of the bond between mother and child, and made furious by the sentimentalizing of it. I know its power, in all its rawness and physicality. That bond was severed for me—not irrevocably, not completely, but daily. My mother returned and left again, returned and left again, staying only for the single hour she was able to visit me.

My mother read me *Ferdinand the Bull, Mike Mulligan and His Steam Shovel, Make Way for Ducklings*. I wanted to hear the same stories over and over again. I waited to hear the words I knew rise up out of the sea of her language: "cork . . . bee . . . matador . . . Ferdinand . . . mallard . . . Mulligan . . . Mary Ann." I didn't want any other books. I didn't want to be surprised by anything, not by clowns leaping out of wind-up boxes that jingle, "Pop Goes the Weasel," not by unfamiliar stories. I wanted my mother's voice to rub away the rough edges of those words, as a river rubs away the rough edges of a rock. I wanted to hold those smooth familiar words against me during the twenty-three hours I had to live through before she would come back to me again.

And then there is my fear of being alone at night.

I have lived in some rough inner-city neighborhoods. Sometimes in Detroit I would hear the distant *pop-pop-pop* of gunfire. Once it came so close that I yelled to my son and his friend, "Get down!" and threw myself on top of them. It's not that I never felt fear, but the fear was always manageable.

I have only felt real terror when I was alone. When I was going to grad school at Stanford, I lived in a suburb for the first time in my life, the kind of place people move to not just for the good schools and ample yards, but for the general air of safety. Sometimes, walking at night to a friend's house a few blocks away, I'd get seized by terror: I'm all alone. I could call out, and no one would hear me. Everyone is shut away in houses set back from the street, behind thick doors.

My worst terror of all came the summer I got the fellowship and lived on the D. H. Lawrence Ranch outside Taos, New Mexico. The property's caretaker was about a quarter of a mile away from my cabin. The next nearest neighbor was five or six miles away. I would be all right until I lay down to sleep. In one part of my mind I knew perfectly well that the noises on the tin roof were squirrels and chipmunks, maybe a raccoon, or maybe pinecones and acorns being blown out of trees, but another part of my mind was convinced someone was out there, and that with no one to hear me scream, no one to come to my aid, I was going to be attacked, murdered in my bed. Once I even called out, "Go away! I've got a gun!"—my empty threat scaring the squirrels on the roof not one whit.

I know I must be recalling the isolation of my first weeks in the hospital. Any sound from another human being—even the *pop-pop* of distant gunfire—is better than the utter desolation of being alone.

"POLIO STRIKES THE MOST FIT . . .
THE MOST BRILLIANT"

I have a memory—surely it can't be right, but nonetheless I have it—of sitting in my hospital crib on Christmas Day in 1954, with presents piled around me. I'm buried in them, up to my neck, as if I'd been buried in sand. I've received a bounty unattainable by other children on the ward with less glamorous afflictions like congenital hip dislocations and scoliosis. I ask my mother about it. She's not sure if I was literally buried up to the neck, but she says, "You got an awful lot of stuff."

I read in the *Mid-York Weekly* that later on, when I returned to the hospital for surgery, the Baptist Sunday School had given me a passel of gifts I'd never received. I got so many presents that my mother had passed some of them along to other kids.

When I was first sick my father would try to pay for a tank of gas only to be told: "It's been taken care of."

When sportswriter Jim Marugg was hospitalized with polio, he received cards, clippings, and jokes from "Everybody on the paper from the publisher down to the newsboys on the streets." Friends and coworkers contributed money:

Men who had families of their own hurried their dinner or skipped it altogether, or gave up their one free evening a week in order to drive Sylvia over to the hospital and wait patiently in the parking lot while she came in for her five-minute visit. Neighbors sat with the children, mowed the lawn, helped with housework, sent in food. . . . Prayers were made for me, votive candles burned before saints.

Many other disabilities—mental illnesses, developmental disabilities, cleft palates—wore a mantle of shame. FDR, as President Franklin Roosevelt was known, played an instrumental role in making polio an illness that made the sufferer less a debased figure and more a heroic victor. He did such a good job of it that Supreme Court Justice William O. Douglas—a god second only to Roosevelt in my parents' liberal pantheon, who has been revealed as a glib liar since his death—apparently cooked up the story that he, too, had had polio and overcome it. Roosevelt understood that he had to create a narrative to counter the expected one about tragedy and loss and shame. He made the story of his disability one of triumph over it, presenting himself as a man who had not just "overcome" his disability but been strengthened by it.

When I was seven or eight years old, an old man stopped me as I was walking near the swan pond on the Colgate campus and asked me the familiar question, "What happened to you, sweetheart?" "I had polio." I suppose he must have said some words of encouragement to me—about doctors, and doing exercises, and getting better, or perhaps praised me for being such a trouper. And then he said, "You know President Roosevelt had polio." I could only think, How could he possibly think I don't know that? But I was too polite—or more likely too stunned—to say, "I know."

Hugh Gallagher's *FDR's Splendid Deception* details the ways that Roosevelt hid the extent of his impairment—having the Secret Service seize film that had been taken while Roosevelt was being lifted; rehearsing the walk he would make to the podium to accept the Democratic Party nomination, a cane in his right hand, one of his sons gripping his other arm, essentially carrying him upright to the podium; being driven to a special stand from which he would throw out the opening ball for the baseball season. And yet the fact that Roosevelt remained disabled was an open secret. During the debate about whether Roosevelt should be depicted in a wheelchair at his memorial in Washington, an April 26, 1997 letter to the *Times* noted that, in the working-class Manhattan neighborhood of the letter writer's boyhood, Roosevelt's opponents talked openly of him as "that cripple in the White House."

In the mid-1940s, at the polio rehabilitation center at Warm Springs, Georgia, writer Bentz Plagemann thought that he found the female patients so beautiful because he had not seen American girls for years, having been in the navy during the war. He mentioned this to his physical therapist, whose name, Miss Plastridge, seems quite apt. " 'But they are beautiful,' Miss Plastridge said. 'You must remember that polio strikes the most fit; the healthiest, the gayest, the most brilliant.' " When he first arrived, she had told him that " 'Only a particular group of people contract polio. . . . It indicates a highly organized central nervous system, which usually means talent, or special ability of some kind."

Not everyone who had polio was embraced by their families and their communities. At a coffee shop in Los Angeles, I strike up a conversation with a burly man—a construction worker or handyman, he has tools hanging from his belt—sitting next to me. He tells me he had polio, too. When he was first sick, the family doctor told his mother, "Put him in the back room and shut the door. Let him go." Peg Kehret, hospitalized in 1949, had four roommates at Sheltering Arms, a rehab hospital in Minneapolis. One of them, Alice, had been abandoned by her parents at the age of three when they realized she would never fully recover from polio. For the previous ten years she had remained in the hospital. When Peg's parents said they were going to bring all the girls presents at their next visit, the other girls asked for marshmallows and licorice and comic books, but Alice was unable to name anything. "Alice had been at Sheltering Arms for so long she didn't remember things like comic books and marshmallows. Licorice and potato chips were beyond her realm of experience."

MILKWEED, CREEKS, AND QUICKSAND

"Apr 55" is stamped at the top of the black-and-white photograph with a white deckled edge, shot with my parents' Brownie Instamatic. Less than a month had passed since I had left the hospital. Four girls, chubby in their snowsuits, are making mud pies on the side porch, stirring mud with wooden spoons in cake pans and tin cans. Only Sandra, a front tooth missing, looks up at the camera: The rest of us are intent on our *pâtisserie de boue*. In another photograph, taken later that same day, we are lined up, sitting on the half wall of the porch. Only if you look closely will you notice that the leg of one of the four sisters is held at an awkward angle, my brace keeping it rigid at the knee.

Once a reporter interviewing me said, "You must have spent your childhood pretty much indoors," and I laughed, because my childhood was so physically expansive. I'm struck by how often media representations of disabled people seem to keep us confined: not just inside buildings, but our bodies themselves contained. One of my least favorite movies of all time is *Extreme Measures*. The plot revolves around the kidnapping of homeless people by an underground alliance between doctors and disabled people, who then force the captives to undergo medical experiments in pursuit of a cure for spinal cord injury. None of the disabled characters in the movie ever *spoke*, at least in the hour or so I endured before I walked out, and they were all virtually frozen in their wheelchairs—a sort of *Night of the Living Dead* meets *Freaks*.

In fact the disabled body is often not contained. It lurches, slouches, has spasms and seizures. Our power wheelchairs disturb the peace in libraries. The containment in which we are so often portrayed seems rather the expression of a deeply held wish: Hold still! Stop it! Be quiet! Stay off the streets! Hide yourself from public sight!

My first happy memory is leaving the hospital to buy a pair of shoes: riding in the front seat of a nurse's car, the smell of the air beyond the hospital walls, the sight of trees and telephone wires rushing past the window, the thrill of being outside.

When I came back from the hospital to the house on East Lake Moraine Road, the house bordered by six maple trees, I returned to a life that was lived mostly outdoors. In the summer I lived in my bathing suit and in the winter in snow pants, boots, hats, earmuffs, mittens, and parkas. My sisters and brother and I built snowmen and, when the snow was particularly densely packed and icy, my father would help us build igloos, cutting the ice and snow into thick blocks that we'd stack into a dome.

Our gray-shingled farmhouse sat on a hundred acres of land, a few acres of which were given over to our vegetable garden and fields that we rented to various neighbors to plant with corn and strawberries. The rest of the land was wild. Mr. Carpenter, who pastured some of his Holsteins on our land, paid his yearly rent by giving us half a slaughtered dairy cow, which my father hung upside down in the woodshed while its blood dripped from it. During the day when it hung there, my sisters and I dared one another other to look. Weak stomached, I always lost those dares. My sisters could also make me vomit by singing, "Great green gobs of/greasy, grimy gopher guts . . ." I wasn't even able to tell on them, because if I tried to say to my mother, "They're singing the 'gopher guts' song," I would start gagging before I could get the word "gopher" out of my mouth. Anyhow, "telling" was looked down on in our family. "Fight your own battles," my parents used to say.

A girl with blond ringlets, the daughter of a farmer, told my sisters and me that she had been spanked only once. Spanked only once? She might as well have told us that she had a golden coach and eight white horses. Once? Really? Only once? We rarely got through dinner without one of us spilling our milk or teasing another one, and then my father would put us across his knee, pull down our pants, and spank us on our bare bottoms.

When our elementary school principal, Mr. Kazaznak—everyone called him Mr. K—saw me on the stairway, he'd scoop me up in his arms and say, "Don't ever go out in the rain. Do you know why? Because sugar melts in the rain—and you are made of sugar."

Mr. English, the brace maker, carried me in his arms, too, down the flight of steps into his basement workshop. He lived on a tree-lined street in Utica. Behind the line of trees was a second line, of triple-decker houses. The houses were all solid upstate rectangles, painted white with brown trim or brown with tan trim. Everything was so much more orderly in those days. The women were in charge of the houses. They bought cake mixes, yellow or chocolate, made by Betty Crocker—or, if they put on airs, Duncan Hines—and squishy white loaves of Wonder Bread (Helps Build Strong Bodies 12 Ways) at the Grand Union. The wives and mothers did their housework in shirtwaist dresses of buttercup yellow or robin's-egg blue or heliotrope. The skirts of their bright dresses twirled around them as, filled with postwar bliss, they pirouetted from the stove to the refrigerator, from the refrigerator to their dining room tables, in their efficient modern kitchens. When they knelt down to sweep their dust piles into dustpans, their skirts spread around them like happy pools of butter left out on a hot day.

Women had dominion over the physical space of their houses. Men were in charge of the rest of the world. They also got the basements of the houses. Sometimes the basements were finished, and then men might have electric train sets down there that sped through plastic tunnels in plastic mountains and past miniature plastic villages; or workshops, like the one where Mr. English made my braces.

The yellow light of Mr. English's basement wasn't the yellow of the women's buttercup dresses or of Betty Crocker cakes: It was the yellow of kerosene lamps and old newspapers. Mr. English had drawers full of leather straps and buckles, he had racks of metal bars that were like the girders of Erector sets—but far sturdier—and tools that hung on corrugated pegboards. Did old braces and leather straps really hang from the ceiling like stalactites? When he was riveting together a joining on my braces, he might nick his finger and say, "Aw, heck." I got scared when men swore, even if it was just "heck."

When Mr. English carried me down the stairs I smelled his smell of cigarettes and maleness and aftershave. Grown-ups always smelled bad to me.

My father's grad students carried me sometimes, too. They called me "Princess." When I look around the seminar table at my own grad students, with their barely postadolescent skin and wispy beards, I know those college students couldn't have been as handsome as I remember them. In the memories of my childhood, Hamilton, New York, is populated by men who are square jawed and rugged and have steel blue eyes, all waiting to gather me up in their strong arms and carry me off.

The rent for the fields where Glen Denmark grew corn and strawberries was paid in kind. "The minute corn is cooked," my mother used to say, "its sugar starts turning to starch." I had a literal image of grains of white sugar and the powdered starch my mother dissolved in an enamel basin and used to stiffen the skirts of our party dresses. My mother would have the water boiling before we picked the corn from the upward sloping field that adjoined our backyard. We were anything but gourmets though. Frugality ruled. At the end of the summer, we'd all gather in the kitchen to shuck corn from the cob so it could be frozen in the special freezer boxes, pale blue with white snowflakes.

My best friend, Debby Brown, and I would hike up past the rusted tiller, slowly being swallowed up by rangy grasses. There were some plants that I hated. Burdocks were the worst, their fruit covered by a ball of barbs that would get caught in our hair and clothes. My mother would have to yank them from my head while I whined and carried on. "It hurts! It hurts!" "—I *know* it hurts, but I have to get it out of your hair." Once or twice she had to resort to cutting my hair in order to free one from my head. I hated the unpruned pear tree next to the chicken coop because a colony of yellowjackets built their mud-and-wattle nest there. To this day, although I like pears when I actually eat them, I still have an instinctive aversion to them, a Pavlovian response to the stings I got from the yellowjackets, far more painful than those of an ordinary bumblebee. I always got a few of the latter during the summer, generally when I was walking across the yard in my bare feet. And I have never been able to bring myself to drink burdock-root tea.

It was the mysterious, single bloodred dot in the midst of the cluster of flowerets that made me love Queen Anne's lace—along with the fact that it had my name. I loved the story that went along with it. The queen had pricked her finger as she wove, and the drop of blood stained the otherwise perfect white filigree. Milkweed was magical, too. At the right time of year you could split the pods open with the pressure from your thumb and, with a puff of breath, send the thousands of seeds, each with its own white silk parachute, flying to the wind. If the pods weren't mature you'd open the sage green pod only to find the filaments weighted down with white slime. Too late, and the seeds would already have flung themselves to the wind, leaving behind the empty husk, fading to brown.

Debby and I would clamber onto the rock pile, where the stones cleared from the adjacent field had been heaped. Every rock we picked up had a fossil in it. Some rocks seemed to be nothing but clusters of fossils—ancient scallops and clams and snails. Others held a single imprint from a trilobite or long-extinct fern. Some of the fossils were almost infinitesimal, only a little bigger than a grain of sand. While we were examining fossils, our attention might be caught by a hammering sound, and we'd look up to see a woodpecker drilling its bill into the tree above us—always disappointing us by not resembling the cartoon character Woody Woodpecker. Doves cooed; cicadas ticked and made their siren calls. We spent hours and hours there, my aluminum crutches flung onto the ground, my right leg, encased in the metal-and-leather brace I wore outside my jeans, held straight out in front of me. The heavy steel-and-leather braces of those days make the British words for them, "irons," seem a far more accurate term.

When I was in my early forties, having gone without braces for decades, I had to start wearing a brace again on my left leg. My knee had developed complications not so much from the aftereffects of polio as from the orthopedic surgery designed to repair my body after polio. This new brace was made of lightweight metal and Velcro. I wore my leather jacket and my new leg brace on the outside of my jeans. I decided I liked the look—it was *Road Warrior*esque. Despite the fact I'm a former militant smoker, now a militant ex-smoker, I considered bumming a Camel from someone and sticking it behind my ear, or maybe even buying a whole pack so I could turn it up inside the sleeve of a black T-shirt, a middle-aged academic's playful riff.

No one in the 1950s brought an ironic sensibility to the choice of garments—or at least no one we knew. Perhaps, in far-off New York City—upstaters, we were always careful to add the "City"—some did, but not here in Hamilton. Riding the school bus in 1956, I watched the high school girls having to press their hands against their voluminous skirts with their tulle petticoats beneath them, so they could make their way down the bus aisle. As they moved past us kindergartners, we whispered to one another, speculating about how they managed to achieve such vastness. "She must have fifteen slips on." I longed to be sixteen and to have such a skirt. Of course, by the time I was sixteen those cinched waists and full skirts had long since disappeared. I wore bell-bottom jeans from the army-navy surplus store and blue work shirts, and a black-and-white anti-war button that said: "No Negotiations! U.S. Out of Vietnam NOW!"

Did I imagine myself wearing those magnificent skirts with my legs encased in metal braces? I don't think I did. When Posey Smith, one of my mother's friends, laughed about a friend of hers who'd had to go down the aisle on crutches, I imagined myself doing the same, transplanting my face onto the picture of my white-gowned mother in her wedding album and adding my crutches. If I were still using crutches when I got married—despite all the assurances about "getting better," in some corner of my brain I must have believed I would be—would my wedding be laughable? How I would bring together my female self and my disabled self was a conundrum.

A rare fossilized dinosaur egg sat in a glass-and-mahogany case at the museum at Colgate, where my father taught. During the day I believed what I had been told, that fossils were inanimate stone, but at night, alone in my bed, I was not so sure. Maybe the dinosaur egg would hatch. The pterodactyl would use its long beak to poke its way out of the shell, just as I had seen baby robins doing. Then it would poke itself free from the artificial shell of glass and mahogany in which it had been encased. Its wings would be sticky with caked albumen, and it would ruffle and flap them dry. And then—tentatively at first, moving with ever-more-confident and stronger swoops—it would emerge from the building and glide above Hamilton, finally coming to rest, clinging to the spire of the Baptist church in town.

That wasn't the worst of my terrors. Sometimes at night I would become overwhelmed by the riddle of eternity. I would lie awake, tormented by the knowledge that I would someday cease to exist, that even if I became a famous writer, whatever immortality I managed to achieve would, in the end, disappear into the void of time. These thoughts would take over my mind; like a Touretter's twitches and involuntary shouts, like the electrical storms in the brains of someone with epilepsy, the thoughts were *of* me but not controlled by me. Anything might trigger them, including the opening of the weekly television series *Ben Casey,* in which Sam Jaffe, playing Dr. Casey's mentor, solemnly intoned, as he drew symbols on a chalkboard: "Man," and a circle with an arrow angling from it; "Woman," a circle with a plus sign beneath it; "Birth," "Death," ending with "Infinity," as he drew a sideways figure eight. Or a movie from Universal Studios, with its opening logo of the earth spinning in space, the word "Universal" circling around it. Or one of the films sometimes shown in school about astronomy, a male narrator intoning "light-years" and "billions and billions of galaxies." I would become depressed by the thought of my own insignificance.

Sometimes at the dinner table my father would talk about a thought experiment in which a monkey, stuck for eternity in a room with a typewriter, randomly typing out words, would occasionally, completely by happenstance, quite unaware of what he was doing, type a word—"cat," or "dog," or perhaps even "antidisestablishmentarianism." At some point this monkey, plunking away on the keys for all eternity, would type out a complete sentence. And at some point the monkey would type a line from Shakespeare. Yes, we would have to agree, that was inevitable. And at some point, the eternally typing monkey would type out *Hamlet.* I knew that everything my father was saying was completely logical. At the same time I felt I was being led into a labyrinth inhabited by something more terrifying than any Minotaur. Not only was my insignificance being proved, but the very insignificance of language itself. Every time my father began to talk this way, I feared another episode of my terrifying repetitive thoughts was going to be triggered.

I never knew when the thoughts would end. Sometimes they would be in my head for months and months, and for all that time I'd have a feeling in my head that was half a headache, half a high-pitched whine, be so tormented by those thoughts that I'd lie awake in bed for hours and hours with them running through my head. Now I realize that some of those obsessions must have been a reliving of the terror I had felt as a child in the hospital, cast alone into a dark and lonely ocean from which I could see no shore.

My father would sing, "Oh, they don't wear pants / in the southern part of France / and the dance they do / it is called the hootchy-koo . . ." We'd sing along for as long as we could before we dissolved into giggles, while my mother, sitting opposite my father at the foot of the table, murmured over and over again, "Jack, no, no."

Years later another disabled woman, one of the first I allowed myself to know, repeated the commonplace utterance that was too often said to her, "You have your mind," adding tersely, "I have a body, too." Did I hear "You have your mind" when I was a child? I am sure I did, both directly and indirectly.

At any rate I knew that I was supposed to make up for my bodily lack with mental agility: I was expected not to be just a smart kid but the smartest. Did that expectation come from without? Or was it internally generated? Both, I think. It was one of those familial assumptions, all the more powerful for being unspoken. One memory of first grade stands out for me with embarrassing clarity. Dennis Seelbach, my competitor for the role of smartest kid in Mrs. Burke's class, stood at the blackboard, squirming, unable to remember how to spell "horse," while I sat extra tall in my chair, gloating, exultant.

Later on during my childhood, in *Voices in Stone*, I would read of Jean-François Champollion, the man who deciphered hieroglyphics. His mother, seriously ill during her pregnancy with him, had turned to the local sorcerer for aid. After having been laid upon a bed of burning herbs and given "a hot infusion and unguents," his mother gave birth to a son. Of course such a story wouldn't be complete without the sorcerer making a prophecy: "From your travail will be born a boy who will be the light of centuries to come."

The very appearance of the baby gave evidence of his being one of the elect. "The little face with its olive tint, two huge black eyes and heavy black curls was curiously oriental. To his amazement the doctor even noticed the yellow cornea, characteristic of the Levantines."

It depressed me to know that at my birth I had revealed no special sign, no Oriental slant to my eyes that hinted at an almost magical genius. No seer had pronounced me special. My mother had spat into the world a baby with a squished head, blotchy vernix-covered skin, blue eyed, ordinary.

Seven of us lived on an assistant professor's salary. Sometimes the tooth fairy left an IOU instead of a dime under our pillows. At the end of the month we might have to lend our parents whatever was left of the weekly allowances they'd doled out to us Saturday mornings in order to come up with the three cents each for our milk money at school. My oldest sister, Sandra, got the new clothes and started them on their downward path. Since everyone around us wore hand-me-downs, we had no sense of deprivation. Recreational shopping was unheard of. My mother substituted it with walks to old farmsteads. On Sunday-afternoon drives, she might spot a rock-lined square hole, the foundation all that was left of a house long since decayed. She collected the old bottles she found there, blue and green and brown blown glass, sometimes with a bubble of air trapped in them, the glassblower's frozen breath. Our own house had a dirt-floored, rock-lined cellar: our house's id. I was afraid to go down there, afraid of the spiders and mice.

Sometimes, on one of these hikes, we'd come across a patch of wild strawberries, miniature versions of the strawberries Glen Denmark cultivated in the field next to our house. The flavor in those cultivated ones seemed to have been diffused and weakened as it spread through the mealy fruit. The wild strawberries were succulent. Surely Adam and Eve, wandering through the Garden, must have come across wild strawberries and hunkered down next to them and eaten them, picking them and popping them into their mouths, just as we did.

I went barefoot all summer long. Seeing me walk on gravel, adults would say, "Doesn't that hurt your feet?" I'd cross my left leg behind my floppy right one so I could lift the right leg up, and then swing myself up on my crutches, momentarily holding both my feet in front of me, proudly displaying the calluses I'd earned over the summer, my feet almost like hooves. I went in the chicken coop to collect eggs in my bare feet. I said I liked the way the mix of sharp straw and squishy chicken shit felt under my feet, but I mostly enjoyed horrifying my mother.

Look magazine showed marines in basic training, crawling under barbed wire. Their muddy faces, shot in high-contrast black-and-white, registered an equal mix of fear and grit, while the caption underneath extolled their bravery. I was singularly unimpressed. We crawled under barbed wire all the time, although our mothers did warn us to be careful around electrified barbed wire, designed to give cattle with wanderlust an extra jolt.

Beyond the six maples, across East Lake Moraine Road, beyond the fields of Glen Denmark's vegetable farm, was a line of willows, and past that the creek that ran along the edge of the Crouches' property. As soon as the snow melted, my younger brother and sister and I would start trooping over to the Crouches' after school and on weekends. The Crouches were like us, a family of five, but not like us. Mr. Crouch was an auto mechanic and sometimes said, "Kiss my ass." We'd walk along the gravel on the side of the road—single file, our mother reminded us, facing traffic.

It would have been shorter to cut across the field, but Debby's older brother told us there was quicksand there. Duncan knew everything—he was in high school and had a ham radio in the closet of his bedroom and would talk to other ham radio operators in Alaska or California. Alaska. California. High school. We believed him when he said melted ice cream turned into poison. We would scarf down the Grand Union brand of vanilla, despite the headaches from eating it so fast. In addition to Duncan's authority, quicksand, like amnesia, was a frequently used plot device on the TV shows Debby and I used to watch on the black-and-white TV in her den. We still didn't have a television, the last family on earth without one. Our favorite show was *The Lone Ranger*, although we also watched *Sky King* and *The Roy Rogers Show*. Characters on those shows were always finding themselves trapped in quicksand, and Debby and I knew the drill. "Don't fight it," Dale or Tonto might say, from the safety of solid ground: "If you struggle you'll just go down faster." Even though I was sure *I'd* be able to get out—I wouldn't panic, I knew better than to struggle—I avoided the patch of land on that side of the brook. I'd seen one too many guest stars disappear with a slurp and final bubble.

The creek next to the Crouches' was so narrow I could plant my crutches in the middle of it and leap across. Everyone else had to wade through the cold water to get to the other side. We spent our time at the creek—we pronounced it "crick"—using tin cans to catch crayfish that looked remarkably like some of their fossilized ancestors. Once David Crouch caught a bass with his bare hands, a feat that earned him bragging rights for months.

I was fascinated by the way willow trees, after being chopped down, sent off new shoots from their stumps. My mother's Blue Willow china showed a Chinese scene—or at least an eighteenth-century English version of a Chinese scene. My mother told us the story that went with it, about a love both true and thwarted. There was the bridge across which the two lovers had escaped; the pagoda where the lovers had taken refuge; here was the curved bridge across which the searchers were moving, carrying their lanterns, searching for the elopers; and here were the two lovers, magically turned into doves, united forever.

A few summers after I came back from the hospital my father and his friends—other junior professors from Colgate—built a pool on the side of our yard so I could swim, since swimming was supposed to have miraculous powers to heal the aftereffects of polio. I remember those men, in the hot summer sun of upstate New York, dressed in khaki pants and sleeveless undershirts, mottled with sweat, swinging pickaxes and wielding shovels. In a vertigo of memory I watch them working, simultaneously the four- or five-year-old I was then—to whom they seemed remote, to have existed almost forever—and the fifty-two-year-old woman I am now, who might feel a surge of attraction for those men, drawn to their flesh glistening with sweat, the swing of their pickaxes, their camaraderie. But they were decades younger than I am now. To those young men I would now be the one who would seem remote, impossibly aged.

The pool was more of a swimming hole than a pool, shaped like an inverted cone, paved with the kind of asphalt highway crews use as a temporary patch for streets. There was no outlet for the water, piped down in a long black hose from the well in the pasture. After the asphalt had been laid down, in place of a roller, we piled into the 1930s Model A my father had bought for ten dollars—or was it twenty?—from one of his students. My father drove slowly up and down the sides of the pool while we hollered in delight and terror. A couple of times during the course of the summer—when the strands of algae had become so thick that the water itself seemed green—my father would drain the pool and scoop out the muck that had accumulated in the bottom. Swimming, of course, did not cure my polio. The miracle, looking back on it, is that none of us got hepatitis from swimming in that stagnant water.

Sundays we went on drives in one of the green station wagons we bought secondhand, or in the Model A. None of our cars had a radio—a car radio was a luxury then—and so we sang: "The Marine Hymn"— "From the halls of Montezuma to the shores of Tripoli . . ." and "The Caissons Go Rolling Along"—"Over hill, over dale, we will hit the dusty trail / As the caissons go rolling along." It wasn't that my family was particularly militaristic: It was just that in the wake of World War II, those were the singalong songs my parents knew. We also sang "Go Down, Moses," the gospel tune that was becoming a civil rights song.

Tree climbing always eluded me. Although my arms were strong, I didn't have the trunk strength to hoist myself into a tree, but I didn't think that I couldn't climb trees—I only thought I hadn't yet figured out the right technique or met the right tree. It turned out to be the latter. When I was ten years old we moved to Providence, where an enormous silver beech with low-hanging branches took up much of our front yard. I could straddle those low branches and shimmy along to the trunk and then work my way to the higher branches.

Years later I had to take a battery of vocational tests in order to get assistance from Massachusetts Vocational Rehabilitation, known as Mass Rehab. (I suppose to the uninitiated Mass Rehab sounds as though it might be either the name of a Catholic liturgical reform movement or a collective drug treatment program.) On one of the tests I had to answer questions like "I would rather go to a football game than watch a ballet," "I would rather work on a crossword puzzle than go to a party." The rehab counselor smiled when she reported the results to me, saying, "We got a very unusual result on this test," because I combined strong intellectual interests with a decided preference for the outdoors. Most times the test came up with a list of possible occupations. For me it indicated only one: park service administrator. Unfortunately, the counselor said, Rehab could not pay to train me for such an occupation, since it would require a graduate degree, and Rehab could only fund occupational plans that were attainable with a bachelor's degree. So my vocational goal, at least to the bureaucracy, was to be a library assistant—which just happened to be the vocational goal for nearly every mobility-impaired female.

"DO SOMETHING! . . . DO ANYTHING!"

Not to act in the face of the crisis of polio was unthinkable. To allow a disease simply to run its course seemed heretical. It is hardly surprising that one researcher later titled his history of polio epidemics in Canada *"Do Something! . . . Do Anything!"* And yet there was relatively little medicine could do to affect the course of an active polio infection. It was mostly a matter of waiting until the infection had coursed through the body. Hot packs might relieve pain—although they were often so hot that they merely substituted one sort of pain for another. If someone's respiratory muscles were in danger of being paralyzed, being put in an iron lung would probably save her life. Once the disease was no longer acute, physical therapy and even surgery were sometimes helpful. But waiting and inaction hardly seemed an appropriate response to the crisis phase of the illness.

"Something" and "anything" were sometimes done to the individual bodies of people with polio and sometimes carried out on the community as a whole. Although there was no evidence that the disease was spread by flies, swatting flies became a way of warding off the disease during the 1916 New York epidemic. In June of that year the *Newark Evening News* ran a drawing of an infant cowering before a hirsute fly—one larger than the child pictured. "No Fairy-Tale Hobgoblin," the title proclaimed, and the text went on:

> I am the Baby-Killer!
> I come from garbage-cans uncovered,

From gutter pools and filth of streets,
From stables and backyards neglected,
Slovenly homes—all manner of unclean places.
I love to crawl on babies' bottles and baby lips;
I love to wipe my poison feet on open food
In stores and markets patronized by fools.

Why the fly? On the most obvious level, flies could be seen while germs could not. The fly theory allowed people to take action. The solutions proposed by the germ theory were negative and essentially static— "Don't let your child go to parties, picnics or outings," read the notice displayed on motion picture screens in New York that summer. "Don't let your children play with any children who have sickness at home. . . . A watched child is a safe child." The fly theory, on the other hand, allowed people to engage in activity to prevent the disease. They could buy screens for their windows. They could swat flies and encourage those around them to do the same. They could organize within their communities to hold fly-swatting contests, to engage in neighborhood cleanups, and to boycott merchants judged to be unsanitary. They could help the poor by providing them with screens and lidded refuse containers.

Since polio was conceptualized as a disease of immigrant filth, the "fly theory" also explained how polio could appear in clean suburban and rural homes. It became part of the mythology that saw the disease spreading outward from "congested" urban areas to the presumably more healthful pastoral areas.

The fly became a carrier, not just of contagion, but of displaced emotions. We need not fear the innocent, suffering child. We could fear the fly instead. We need not feel our fear of and even rage toward those who were simultaneously sick and carriers of infection. We could kill the fly. The fly was ugly, it was hairy, it was dark, it was Other.

The "anything" that had to be done was also done to the bodies of those with the disease. "Vapor Tried on Patients" read a headline in the *World* on August 29, 1916. At New York's Willard Parker Hospital, children were tied into frames, with the hopes of preventing deformities. Faradism—the name was adapted from that of the British scientist Michael Faraday, a means of causing a mild muscular contraction through electrical stimulation—was also used. Vermont's Dr. Caverly described it as "disagreeable, and to young children often a source of terror." Over the years patients came to be injected with the smallpox vaccine; adrenaline; serums derived from horses, sheep, goats, and monkeys; as well as serums made from the blood of those who had recovered from the disease. The variability of polio—the fact that sometimes the disease receded, leaving very little damage in its wake, or that return of function could occur after an initial bout of paralysis, meant that remedies might appear to be effective when the apparent cure was due only to the vagaries of the disease. Wanting to help, wanting to act, those caring for people with polio sometimes painted the bodies of their patients with hot wax; had them dipped repeatedly in hot water, then in cold seawater; anesthetized patients and pounded their muscles with rubber mallets; and rubbed them down with goose grease. At least one polio patient had his already paralyzed muscles injected with curare, the paralytic poison into which the indigenous people of the Amazon dip their arrows. When the patient later questioned a doctor who had not been involved in this treatment what the reason for it had been, he was told, "Well, it gave them something to do." During the period when prolonged splinting was employed, some patients were immobilized for months or even years. Ultimately most of these treatments had little effect on the disease, and some, particularly complete immobilization, worsened its aftereffects.

In New York in the summer of 1916, those who had had infantile paralysis in previous epidemics were recruited to donate their blood so that serum could be made from it. This was yet another ineffective treatment. *The World* gave not only the names and addresses of five of the eight who had donated blood for serum at a local hospital but also the number of ounces of blood obtained from each—David Jacobs, aged forty-three, gave ten ounces, while from the youngest donor listed, nine-year-old Ida Loomer, only an ounce and a half was drawn.

Almost from the start there was controversy over medical actions. On August 2, 1916, *The World* informed its readers that "Doctors Dispute Over Treatments as Plague Grows: Dr. Bermingham of Throat Hospital Calls Serum's Use Ridiculous and Suggests Preparation Made from a Rabbit Shot in a Graveyard." The accompanying article further amplified Dr. Bermingham's suggestion by revealing that he had suggested, tongue firmly in cheek, that "the serum should be made from the blood of a jack rabbit, killed by the light of the moon in a graveyard at midnight by a one-eyed [*sic*] negro."

Surgery was another means of "doing something" for people who'd had polio. Our ankles and spines were fused into immobility. Muscles and tendons were transplanted. Staples were put into the knees of our "good" legs to keep them from growing faster than our "bad" legs. Sometimes a vein was run from our hearts to our weaker legs to encourage growth.

I had my first operation the summer I was six years old, with a second one later that summer. My mother had attempted to prepare me for it by getting me a children's book about a boy who has his tonsils out. Johnny goes to sleep, and when he wakes up, Mommy is waiting there, and his throat is a little bit sore, but he has ice cream and goes home, with the smiling nurses and doctors waving good-bye to him.

The gruesome fairy tales of the brothers Grimm would have been better preparation. There are certain words that evoke in me a mix of fear and disgust and loneliness: "Gurney . . . ether . . . operation . . . Utica." If it were possible to kill words, I would murder these. And I wouldn't allow them anything approaching a peaceful death, no remote and orderly execution. I would choke them to death, throttle them, put my hands around them and squeeze the life out of them. I would take pleasure in their death throes, their struggle to live. A moment of perverse satisfaction: Someday this English language will have become extinct, a dead, forgotten tongue, and those words will have died with it.

My memories of my first surgery are potsherds, retrieved from the earth. There are gaps in my memory, but enough shards remain that I can lay them out in a rough shape that shows the form of the original whole. Nearly half a century later, I have memories of the morning I first had surgery that are more acute than my memories of yesterday morning. For instance, I remember the smell and feel of the ancient brown leather covering the thin mattress set upon the wheeled gurney to which I was transferred. It was covered with a white cotton sheet, but at some point, either because the sheet was disturbed in my transferring to the wheeled stretcher or because the sheet was too short and failed to cover it completely, I saw the leather itself. The leather had become mottled with use, and deep creases veined it, so it almost appeared to have become a living thing. Beneath a thin veneer of disinfectant scent was a smell of body odors: the acrid smell of someone else's fear, the baser and even more frightening smell of shit and blood that came from deep within the body. Like the sheet on my hospital bed, the sheet laid across the gurney was stiff. Stenciled on the bottom edge of the sheets in black permanent ink were the words "Utica Children's Hospital, Utica, New York."

The nurse who picked me up in her arms and laid me on the gurney had done this hundreds, perhaps thousands, of times before. Maybe the nurse was kind and allowed her hand to rest on my forehead for a few extra seconds. Maybe she smiled at me, told me everything was going to be all right, told me to be good and brave. Still, for her, all these sounds of the hospital—the clatter of the hard rubber wheels of the wheeled stretcher against the linoleum floor, the echo of that clatter off the walls of the corridor, the squeaking of her rubber-soled shoes on the floor— were ordinary sounds, as was the soft, plaintive groan the elevator gave off as its doors parted to admit us. The gulf between how ordinary everything was to her and how terrifying it was to me was enormous.

Even if she was kind, her kindness and comfort would have evoked for me the fact that she was not my mother, the woman who did not need to try to reach me with her kindness, the woman who simply was comfort. The touch of the nurse's hand did not feel like the touch of my mother's hand; the smell of the nurse's body was not the smell of my mother's body.

I was wheeled down the hallway to an elevator. Was the elevator an automatic one, or did it still have an elevator operator, a man or woman perched on a stool whose job it was to push a lever that opened or closed the doors? I don't remember. I'll imagine it had not yet been automated, that a black man looked at me on the stretcher and as he shut the door said, "Basement?" in a gravelly Deep South voice. From the second floor we went down without stopping, passing the first. On the first floor there were the offices, strange places of distant officialdom; the gift shop; the stairs leading to the glass-and-metal front door; the physical therapy rooms, with the pool and the whirlpools and the inspirational sayings on plaques on the wall; the gift shop that sold, along with magazines and cigarettes, crafts that had been made by young women who lived in the hospital: wooden salad bowls with cheerful red-and-yellow designs painted by a paintbrush held in the mouth. On that same first floor, down one of the corridors, lived those who made those gimcracks sold in the gift shop; at least one of whom was in an iron lung. Once, I was taken to visit one of those girls, who remembered me fondly from when I'd first been hospitalized; but when I saw her—a head sticking out of an enormous tank-like contraption—I began to whimper in fear and cling to my mother, as both she and the woman in the lung tried to reassure me.

But now I was being taken down beneath that familiar floor, which, even if it held terrors, held familiar terrors. The operator slowed the elevator as we approached the basement; and then, as we drew closer, eased it down even more slowly, finally stopping it with a quick, decisive lurch: There was an art to this in the preautomatic elevator days.

The elevator operator must have leaned forward, grasped the metal handle of the gate, which folded back onto itself in a series of deft, scissoring motions, rattling as it did so; and then the outer doors must have once again given off their pneumatic sigh as they eased themselves open. The basement was nothing like the upper floors of the hospital, with their bright fluorescent lights and linoleum. In older buildings that were constructed before disability-access codes took effect and have cobbled-together accessible routes, I sometimes enjoy wheeling through the nonpublic spaces of buildings, the glimpse, say, in a fancy hotel, of the life beneath that makes the glittering life above possible: the vast wheeled carts with canvas sides holding bales of white linen, the sharp smells of detergent, the clatter of glassware and pots and pans, the clouds of steam issuing from a dishwashing room.

When I was six years old a basement was a cellar was a dungeon was a black hole. The Christian hell, the Greek Hades, the Norse underworld: They were all places buried deep within the earth. I was being wheeled along a corridor that ran between the children's hospital and the big hospital that abutted it. Exposed pipes ran overhead, painted with dark brown paint that served no decorative purpose but was merely to protect the pipes from corrosion. Here and there were red valves, like the one outside our house that controlled the flow of water to the garden hose, but much larger. At other places the pipes were fitted with various valves and clamps. Pipe, tube, main. Spigot, nozzle, conduit. I know those words now, but as a six-year-old child I did not. Now I know that the naked pipes and tubes and hanks of electrical wiring were carrying water and heat and power to the hospital, and waste away; but then they seemed as strange and unknowable as the glimpsed appurtenances that dangled beneath my father's and my brother's bellies, as the mysterious crevice between my own legs. The namelessness of those objects. My utter incomprehension of what they were for. I opened my eyes, I had to look. I closed my eyes, I couldn't look. I clenched my eyes shut as I was wheeled down that long, terrifying corridor.

I entered the operating room. I was aware, through my closed eyelids, of the brightness of the room. My eyes opened and saw row upon row of lidded jars. I was transferred onto the cold metal table and saw a light fixture above me. It was on a swinging arm, and the light fixture itself was made up of many hexagonal shapes. A few years later, a television Walt Disney nature special showing the structure of a bee's eye—made of multiplying hexagonals—would remind me of that operating-room light and so frighten me that I ran from the room.

The ether mask, lowered down over my face, made the whole world go black. The sharp smell of the gas coiled into the back of my throat, the smell becoming a taste. The world began to spin, like a record on a turntable. As I swirled down into unconsciousness, I flailed my arms and legs while the nurses restrained me.

And then, without any sense of time having passed, I awoke. My mother was next to me, but something had happened to her, too. Her mouth had been replaced by a row of mouths, each one wearing her bright red lipstick, stretching up her face.

"Why do you have so many mouths?"

"It just looks that way," she reassured me. "From the ether."

I went under again—the sensation was more like that of drowning than of falling asleep. When I came awake again, I again asked my mother, "Why do you have so many mouths?"

She held my hand and told me again it was from the ether. As soon as she said those words, I realized, with a sense of confusion and shame that I had asked her that question before, and had gotten the same answer.

"I feel sick."

"Do you think you're going to upchuck?" she asked, and moved to get a curved metal basin, the same kind used in the hospital to spit into when I brushed my teeth.

What I threw up was slimy and thin. I had almost nothing in my stomach. I began to cry. I knew that another surgery was planned for later that summer, and I pleaded with my mother: "Mommy, don't make me have another operation."

My mother soothed me, and I was pulled back down once more into the thick chemical stupor.

Once again, when I came to, my mother's face was distorted. Once again I asked her what had happened to her.

And she repeated to me that nothing was wrong with her face, it was the ether. As soon as she said that, the realization that I had asked that question, and been given that same answer, over and over again snapped into place, and with it a sense of embarrassment and strangeness. I must have been in pain, but I have no recollection of that. Instead what I recall is the way the very foundation of the world seemed to have been shaken: my mother's distorted face, the sure division between being awake and being asleep.

Again I begged her, "Please don't make me have another operation."

"Don't think about that now, sweetie."

But it was all I could think about.

"Please," I begged. My grandmother had set aside one hundred dollars for each of us when we were born, and I knew that this one hundred dollars was waiting for me in a bank account. "Please. Don't make me have another operation. I'll give you a hundred dollars. Please."

"Don't think about that now," she said.

I fell under again, but the anesthesia was beginning to wear off, and when I woke up again, I began to plead with her. "Please, don't make me have another operation. I'll give you a hundred dollars. I'll give you a hundred dollars."

Later, when the anesthesia had worn off, I remembered having flailed at the nurses as I went under. In my mind I had kicked the nurses, and I was afraid that my parents were going to be told of this. Would my father come to the hospital and yell at me and spank me for having kicked the nurse? Since I was regularly reprimanded and spanked for crying, it did not seem at all unlikely.

In the early 1950s Nadina LaSpina contracted polio in the Sicilian village of Riposto. Among the initial treatments she received was electrical shock to the spine—one of the many bizarre applications of electricity in an attempt to stimulate nerves. When that failed her father took her to the mainland, to Rome and to Bologna, seeking, if not a complete cure for her, a way for her to walk. Eventually he became convinced that in America she would walk. One of her father's brothers, already in the United

States, provided a foothold. After their hopes had been raised and dashed numerous times, the family was finally able to emigrate.

Once here they began a round of surgeries—seventeen in all—each of which seemed to offer the elusive promise of walking. Muscles were moved; tendons were stretched; finally her spine itself was fused, and she lay immobilized in a body cast for more than a year. Nadina and her family, like the gambler who believes that his string of losses assure a big win on the next hand, believed the next surgery would be the one that would enable her to walk. At last she did walk—on crutches, with braces—but walking presented its own series of problems. She fell often, falls so severe that they resulted in broken bones. Finally, in her twenties, it seemed that the only way she would be able to continue walking would be to have her lower legs amputated and fitted with prostheses. That was the last of her surgeries. "After that, I realized—I'm not going to torture this body anymore."

When I was in my twenties, a woman I knew had a knee ailment. She was telling a group of us about it, and mentioned that surgery was one of the possibilities she was considering. Someone else in the group said, "Oh, no surgery!" This was the early seventies, and the general belief was that acupuncture and brown rice would cure all ills.

"People say that—oh, no, not surgery—but I feel like if I have surgery, the underlying problem will get fixed," the woman with the knee ailment said.

I would have been less shocked if she had said she thought the world was flat. It had never occurred to me that surgery could actually correct a problem. Surgery seemed an instrument of humiliation, a strange and irrational ritual of degradation.

THE KENNY TREATMENT

By the time I had polio, the treatment of choice in the acute stage was a technique known as "hot packing," developed by a nurse, Elizabeth Kenny, as a treatment in the Australian outback. It involved soaking torn-up wool blankets in boiling-hot water, wringing them out, and applying them to the muscles affected by polio. I have no memory of the treatment; but Charles Mee certainly does: "It was such a bizarre, disgusting procedure that no one who had polio in those days has forgotten what seemed like punishment for having gotten sick."

Mee, like so many others, recalls the hot packs that at first burned one's skin but soon cooled and became clammy. For many of us, "the smell of wet wool possesses almost hallucinogenic powers." I have always hated that smell and break out in a rash when wool touches my body. Even knitting with wool yarn brings on an asthma attack.

While some people found that hot packs relieved them of pain, others found the treatments themselves painful: "Two times every day the therapists took hot packs out of the boiling water. The wool was too hot for them to touch so they used tongs. Every time they threw them on my bare legs I screamed."

Following polio, many muscles were left tight and rigid. It made sense to use heat in order to relax them, but why did the hot packs have to be so hot that they burned the flesh? Why was it essential that they were made of itchy wool? Wouldn't cotton or linen have been more benign? To answer those questions, we need to look at the history of Sister

Elizabeth Kenny, one of the most fascinating characters in the history of polio.

Sister Kenny wasn't a nun, but an Australian nurse who claimed to have found a revolutionary treatment for polio. In polls in the 1940s, she was the second most admired woman in America—Eleanor Roosevelt was the first. In 1952 she came in ahead of Mrs. Roosevelt. The other women who made the list of most admired women in America were either wives of prominent men or movie stars. Elizabeth Kenny was alone in gaining a place on the list as an independent, self-directed woman.

Sister Kenny's descent from fame can be tracked in the pale blue checkout slip glued to the end leaf of the copy of her autobiography, which I checked out from the UC Berkeley Library. Throughout the 1940s and early 1950s, there's a flurry of due dates stamped in purple and blue ink. Then *And They Shall Walk* is left on the shelf for twenty-five years, and finally dispatched to the storage facility—a mysterious place, I imagine it windowless and bunkerlike, in East Oakland, maybe—whence it had to be specially recalled.

Sister Kenny, like polio, had faded out of our collective memories, becoming a footnote to a disease that had itself become a footnote.

The story of Elizabeth Kenny, as told in the 1946 movie version of her life and in her autobiography, is the story of a noble crusader, a solitary and scorned bearer of the truth. Just glancing over Kenny's *And They Shall Walk* gives an idea of the near-religious fervor with which she approached what she called "The Work." Indeed, she sometimes said she was "God's instrument." From its dedication "To the Mothers of Mankind" to her chapter titles ("The Battle Is Joined," "Eyes Have They but They See Not . . . ," ". . . Ears but They Hear Not," "A King, a Prince, and a Little Child," "Hail, America," "The End Crowns All") one senses that she is a woman on a mission, and woe unto her or him who stands in her way. (One article about Kenny had the title "God Is My Doctor.")

Even the appendixes of her life story, which one might expect would carry technical information about her treatment methods or summaries of clinical studies, instead contain treacly paeans to her: "My meeting with Sister Kenny was one of those happy events that occasionally fall like manna from heaven upon the deserving and the undeserving alike." "The world laughed at Robert Fulton, at Thomas Edison, at Louis Pasteur, and the world laughed at Sister Kenny." "To the casual eye, this gathering might look like thousands of similar ones—a luncheon in honor of a celebrity. . . . But this occasion is unique, because we are not honoring *anyone*—instead we are being honored by the presence of a woman who has given the United States of America—and all the world—something which is literally priceless." Clearly this was a woman who had no truck with false modesty. She was also someone who didn't let a little thing like the truth get in the way of a good story.

Elizabeth Kenny was an imposing figure, described as carrying herself "like a queen," as being "an Amazon in white," or as looking "like a good blocking back at Notre Dame." Above those gridiron shoulders she wore hats so distinctive that for a while they were put on display at the institute that bears her name in Minneapolis, a collection of always dark, always ornate, always massive toppers that often paid homage to her native Australia—perhaps by having an emu's plume at a jaunty angle, or emulating an Australian digger's hat, with its distinctive upturned brim.

In New York City policemen sometimes recognized her by her imposing headgear and stopped traffic for her. She was the sort of woman who said to the driver from the backseat of a car, "I like to go fast and by all means do not crawl along for my benefit." Her nurse trainees nicknamed her the Iron Horse. One of them remembered her as "a person who sapped every ounce of energy out of you. . . . She also sort of wanted to rule your life."

Kenny was born in Australia in 1880. She later found it convenient to lop six years off her life, giving the date as 1886. Her mother had among her ancestors a convict—an Irishman "transported," as involuntary exile was called, to Australia for stealing a horse—a fact Kenny never divulged during her life. Her father, Michael Kenny, an immigrant from Ireland's county Kilkenny, was a homesteader. One of Michael Kenny's relatives commented drily that "he would have made a good millionaire." Not finding himself in that station of life, however, he seems to have had a rather hard time wresting a living from the earth. The family usually lived in rough cabins of two or three rooms with outer walls and roofs covered with bark, and the interior walls lined with calico or paper. Like all farmers, the Kenny family's life was governed by the weather. Several seasons of excessive rain brought ruin to the family, turning "the clover fields into bogs and ugly quagmires" and devastating the sheep, which they had switched to raising when cattle ranching proved unsuccessful, with "foot rot and fluke."

The family moved often—from Spring Vale to Inverell, from Inverell to Bannockburn, from Bannockburn to Warialda, and from there on to Wallangarra, Ashford, and Nullamanna. A critical reading of Kenny's autobiography, with its almost total omission of any discussion of her father, suggests a difficult relationship between father and daughter. Family dysfunction was not then considered a fit subject for conversation or for the printed page.

Elizabeth Kenny's mother shepherded her family through the moves, cooking over an open fire, making the clothing her family wore, planting vegetable and flower gardens.

In 1946 RKO released a biopic, *Sister Kenny,* starring a miscast Rosalind Russell in the title role. (One of Kenny's patients commented that W. C. Fields would have looked more the part.) The movie opens with Kenny's return to her parents' homestead from nursing school. In fact her formal education seems to have stopped at about sixth grade, after she attended a one-room school. Such limited education was not unusual among rural families in Australia then. Kenny was fortunate in having a mother who considered reading aloud to her children part of her duties. They heard Shakespeare, the Bible, and other works of literature. Furthermore she was growing up in a time and place in which a preliterate, oral culture was alive. Knowledge was passed down and around within communal and familial structures. Even medical care was most often delivered by nonprofessionals. Looking back on her early days in Australia, Kenny said, "Real doctors were few . . . [and these were] assisted by a hardworking band of two-fisted women called the bush nurses." The remoteness of Australian homesteads meant that families cared for their own, perhaps with the help of a neighbor who had become adept at nursing through experience— often long and hard experience. When Kenny herself had pneumonia as a child, her mother treated her by boiling eucalyptus leaves so the fumes would help her to breathe. The clashes Kenny would later have with the medical profession had many roots. Among them were the class and cultural divides between, on the one hand, the professionalized academics, drawn from the upper middle classes, reliant on knowledge learned from books and from association with other professionals, and, on the other, the folk wisdom of the rugged farmers of the Australian outback.

In her autobiography Kenny claims to have trained at a "private hospital" at which she spent three years. There are no details given about the hospital, no anecdotes from her days of training. It's not hard to read the quick gloss as a lie. Victor Cohn, a Minneapolis journalist who wrote a thorough and well-researched biography of Kenny, was never able to find any evidence of her attendance at a nursing school.

When she excised six years from her autobiography, claiming to have been born in 1886 rather than 1880, one of her motives was the knowledge that to be a woman approaching late middle age was to be a woman considered ready for the rocking chair. Perhaps she also wanted to do away with some of those years when her life had been stuck in the doldrums. The idea of being a nurse hit her when she was in her thirties and she declared herself to be one, got a nurse's uniform sewn for herself—the most prominent feature of which was a red nightingale, or short cape—and rode off into the Never-Never, the Australian outback, where your neighbor might do you the favor of performing an appendectomy with a jackknife and where a bush nurse might find herself up to her elbows in birth slime after the woman of the house had farrowed.

In her autobiography Kenny gave an account of the event that was to prove pivotal in her life. Called to a remote cottage, she found a two-year-old girl sick with fever, in pain, lying on a cot with her legs contracted toward her chest. Completely unfamiliar with what was ailing the child, she sent a telegram describing the symptoms to Dr. Aeneas McDonnell, whom she had known since she was a child. While she awaited his reply, the father of another family came to her with the news that two of his seven children were also suffering from what he described as "cow disease." They had been lame for several days, and now neither of them could stand or walk. In all a total of six children in the area were to come down with this strange illness.

At last Kenny received a response to her telegram: "Infantile paralysis. No known treatment. Do the best you can with the symptoms presenting themselves."

Returning to the bedside of her first patient, she realized that heat would help relax the muscles and prevent contractures and deformity. She tried various means of administering heat, which proved unsuccessful for one reason or another. Then:

> At last I tore a blanket made from soft Australian wool into suitable strips and wrung them out of boiling water. These I wrapped gently around the poor, tortured muscles. The whimpering of the child ceased almost immediately, and after a few more applications her eyes closed slowly and she fell asleep.
>
> O sleep, O gentle sleep, I thought gratefully, Nature's soft nurse!
>
> After a short while, however, the little slumberer awoke fretfully and cried out, "I want them rags that wells my legs!"

Hot packs were one part of the Kenny treatment. Kenny believed that muscles weren't paralyzed as a result of polio but were in spasm. She further believed that when the acute stage ended, muscles had become alienated, rather than paralyzed, and needed to be reeducated. None of these terms were conventional medical ones, and Kenny was sometimes greeted with laughter when she used them with doctors.

Although her methods of treatment actually evolved over decades, in the film they are shown as being developed with her very first case. When Dory, the young patient, is told to sit up, she finds she cannot.

"What's the matter, dear?" Rosalind Russell asks. "Don't you want to sit up?"

"I've forgotten how," Dory says. With a little bit of her "reeducation," Sister Kenny soon has Dory "jumping around like a kangaroo."

According to her autobiography, when Kenny again saw Dr. McDonnell, she informed him that all of her patients had recovered. He expressed astonishment that her untutored methods had been so successful. Given that in many cases the initial paralysis recedes leaving no evident loss of motor function, luck could have been responsible for this initial rate of cure.

She claimed that Dr. McDonnell then said, "The way before you is going to be long and hard. . . . You are going to know heartbreak and humiliation. Sorrow will be your lot from this day forward. But if you have the courage to carry on, a great reward will be yours. The great cities of the earth will bid you welcome."

Those who knew the dour Dr. McDonnell had a hard time imagining him uttering those words. At another point Kenny reported that Dr. McDonnell had said:

> You have made a great medical discovery to the medical world. Your spirit shall be crushed and your heart shall be broken, but I am asking one thing of you: never desert the duly qualified medical practitioner. Remember that the duly qualified medical practitioner is the keeper of the nation's health and well-being, and the time will come when that particular department of medicine will ask you to present your findings and recognize you as a contributor to medical science.

Even harder to imagine as an *ex tempore* comment.

In the film Dr. McDonnell takes Kenny to see a room filled with disabled children on crutches and in braces and, as doleful music plays in the background, tells her, "Eighty-eight out of one hundred cases finish this way." His statement was a great exaggeration, as most of the children shown in the film have quite serious impairments.

Sister Kenny certainly had a reputation for working miracles. When Noreen Linduska was hospitalized with polio, working slowly and painfully through rehab, she received a newspaper clipping about Kenny's work from a friend:

> I could almost hear soft organ music playing quietly in the twilight, and see pink and golden clouds on the horizon, as I read of Sister Kenny slowly walking toward a hospital cot on which lay a victim of infantile paralysis—horribly deformed—utterly distracted with unbearable pain. As she arrived at the side of the cot—she raised her hands Heavenward, said something softly to herself, and then brushed her fingers lightly over the afflicted muscles of the unfortunate child before her. And lo! the legs which hadn't a flicker of movement in ten years slowly moved off the cot, and the boy walked!

Even some of Kenny's great successes—and there were some—didn't live up to the myth. When Elizabeth Kenny came to Minnesota in the early 1940s, Dr. John Pohl was one of the local orthopedists who initially approached her with a good deal of skepticism. One of his patients, Henry Haverstock Jr., had received the usual medical treatment of immobilization and splints. After that he'd gone to the polio treatment center Roosevelt had established at Warm Springs, Georgia, where he had received standard physiotherapy. He was fitted with two leg braces, a body corset, and an arm splint. Still he could not even sit up and spent his days lying in bed. Pohl brought Sister Kenny to Haverstock's home. She entered his bedroom and proceeded to pull from her enormous black purse a sheaf of letters that attested to the success of her methods. She read aloud from them until she was persuaded that results might be far more effective than testimonials.

Pohl, doubtful but willing to give Kenny's methods a try, arranged to have Haverstock admitted to Abbott Hospital, where he was treated first with heat, then with movement. Haverstock later recalled that she was "too optimistic"—promising him that he would be "better than normal." Some of his muscles were completely paralyzed, but others were just weakened and responded to Kenny's unorthodox "muscle reeducation." Within a year he left the hospital, walking with crutches. In the spring of 1942 he entered the University of Minnesota and went on to become a highly regarded lawyer, running for Minnesota attorney general and working to remove architectural barriers that made buildings inaccessible to people with disabilities. More than half a century later, when I spoke with him on the telephone, his voice warmed whenever he spoke of Kenny: "All her patients just loved her, and that included me. . . . I revered her."

Although Sister Kenny's treatment had no doubt changed his life, he remained disabled. Probably, in physical appearance, he was closer to the braced and crutch-walking children of the film than to little Dory, hopping about like a kangaroo. The reality was that many of Sister Kenny's patients were left with significant impairments, even if this fact tended to be left out of publicity about her, where it seemed that her patients all but leaped up from their hospital beds and pirouetted across the floor.

In order to understand the successes and failures of the Kenny treatment, we need to look at the medical practices then used in treating polio:

> Doctors, seeing their patients' twisted necks, spines, hips, knees, legs, and feet, their weak and useless "flail" joints, their grotesque combinations of body misalignment and distortion, thus acted by what seemed to be impeccable logic . . . the affected parts had to be held straight to prevent as much distortion as possible, while rest helped heal the spinal cord.

Patients' limbs—sometimes their entire bodies—were immobilized, for weeks, months, even years—strapped to wooden or wire splints or encased in plaster casts. One Australian patient's entire body was encased in casts and a boned corset, with a padlock at the neck to keep her from removing it. "We did not feel 'sick,' " she later recalled. "We simply could not move anymore because we were chained. What was the meaning of those shackles?"

Since any kind of touch is painful during the acute stage of polio, splinting is an agonizing procedure. Robert C. Huse remembers having his limbs splinted during his initial bout with polio and screaming with pain, begging his mother to take the splints off. His mother, although she sobbed along with him, explained through her tears that his body must be kept straight.

Later Huse was hospitalized so that his scoliosis could be straightened. He recalled being taken to "a place called the cast room" where he underwent what reads like a version of medieval torture. After he had been seated on a contraption that looked like a bicycle without wheels, leather straps were brought down from the ceiling,

> . . . and what resembled a dog's muzzle was placed over my mouth. . . . Somewhere in the back of me a pulley was turned and I felt myself being raised up by the neck. My teeth sank into my lower lip and blood dribbled from the corners of my mouth. About the time I thought my head would be separated from the rest of me, the pulley stopped. . . . They worked quickly now, wrapping my trunk in strips of gauze dipped in plaster of Paris from just under my arms down around my chest, stomach and hips. As the wet plaster added more weight to my body my teeth sank deeper into my lower lip, and my head felt as if it were going to explode.

In addition to the physical pain—and psychological torment—such splinting caused, immobilization could also contribute to muscle weakness. Since the polio infection's path through the spinal column can be erratic, some muscles are left with no function while others are weakened but still have some strength. Splinting's complete immobilization of limbs caused even initially undamaged muscles to weaken and even atrophy from disuse.

During a polio epidemic in Los Angeles, 140 nurses were themselves admitted as polio patients at Los Angeles General Hospital. Although all of them exhibited classical polio symptoms of fatigue and weakness, none of them had polio. Their symptoms were probably the result of treatment. Speaking of the atmosphere that prevailed in hospitals during epidemics, one physician said:

> We had to spell each other so that we could go to sleep for four to six hours. It was like being in combat. You have to be on the ball and ready to go all the time. You were tired, exhausted, and frightened at the same time. We didn't want to get polio ourselves. . . . Nobody had any hours off; it was just taboo. In fact, your colleagues would be really angry. . . . we all lost a lot of weight. Some of the residents and interns I was with were almost cracked up over it.

One can easily imagine how panic would spread. Not surprisingly the overworked nurses would have had sore muscles; the exhaustion they surely must have felt would have translated into fatigue. In the atmosphere of fear and heightened sensitivity to the possible spread of polio, these symptoms caused great concern:

> The nurses were left to the earnest ministrations of a group of young interns who felt it their duty to give them especially good care since they were in a sense colleagues. Accordingly, when the nurses started streaming into the hospital as patients, the young doctors followed the current method of treatment for paralytic poliomyelitis with more enthusiasm than discretion. They immediately applied plaster casts and sometimes erected a frame over the bed, equipped with ropes and pulleys . . . prompt immobilization sometimes for long periods of time made the evaluation of muscle weakness difficult.

Anyone who has ever spent a few days in bed after surgery or during an illness knows how swiftly muscle weakness can set in. Imagine how weak these nurses, encased in plaster and rigged up to elaborate traction, must have become. The symptoms of a disease were produced by the method of treating it.

Sister Kenny's contention that splinting harmed patients was at first considered medical heresy. Quite quickly, however, that part of her treatment became standard practice. In the late 1940s the National Foundation for Infantile Paralysis sold thousands of the splints it had stored for use in epidemics. A farmer near Warm Springs bought some. They were seen in his fields, stuck in the earth, with the leaves and tendrils of his pole beans twisting around them. Doctors seemed to have "forgotten they ever employed prolonged immobilization."

The attitude that use of orthopedic equipment marks whether or not someone is really disabled explains some of Sister Kenny's claims that her methods of treatment rescued her patients from the fate of being "cripples." Part of Kenny's "unmaking" of cripples was that she urged her patients to get around without stigmatized devices—braces, crutches, wheelchairs, and canes.

Call it the Law of Orthopedic Appliances: When I'm in my wheelchair I'm really quite mobile and independent: I sail along, push doors open with my footrests, can carry what I need to, either cradled in my free left arm (my right hand being on the joystick) or slung in a canvas bag over the back of the chair. In this situation offers of help are frequent. When I'm walking on crutches—which I still do occasionally, although less and less often these days—I get far fewer offers of help, although, since walking on crutches is far more difficult, it's a situation in which I more often do need help. People assume that, since I'm walking on crutches—a step down in the hierarchy of orthopedic equipment—I'm therefore *less disabled.*

Speaking of one of her first American patients—almost certainly Henry Haverstock, although she does not use his name—Kenny wrote: "He received eleven months of the best orthodox treatment in the United States of America, and he was a helpless cripple. He is now practicing law and is able to get about and live the life of a useful citizen. He is certainly not one hundred percent recovered, but he is not a cripple." Given that he remained significantly impaired, what was it that made him "not a cripple"?

In *No Time for Tears,* published in 1952 (and given the imprimatur of a foreword by Eleanor Roosevelt and an introduction by then-governor of California, Earl Warren), the father of Chuck (a "polio," as the text has it) states the problem succinctly: "It boils down to solving a big problem: is your child going to grow into a normal human, or is he headed toward miserable years of self-pity and neuroticism?" Addressing himself explicitly to other parents of children with "crippling diseases," he promises that "this story of the actual polio experience" will show "a parent's part in guiding a child away from neuroticism and self-pity." Clearly one part of the answer is that being a cripple is not just a physical state. If one falls prey to neuroticism (a psychological failure) or self-pity (a moral weakness), one will have failed to reach the Holy Grail of "a normal life."

In the movie *Sister Kenny*, Dr. McDonnell says of the children whom medicine has not cured that they will be "hidden away in little houses in forgotten streets with brokenhearted parents."

Being crippled, then, is a state of soul and mind, not just a state of the body. Cripples do not live "normal" lives. They do not attend schools and colleges designed for nondisabled people. Their lot in life is to remain hidden. They are lost in a wilderness of self-pity and neuroticism, for it is not just the body that is bent in crippledom, but the soul and the psyche that twist in concert with the body.

In treating the polio survivor as someone who would be rehabilitated—come hell or high water—Kenny fostered the attitude that her patients would be reintegrated into the world they had been part of prior to their illness. In July 1946 Dr. John Pohl reported: "In six years we have treated 500 Minneapolis polio victims, and not a single one is in a crippled children's school or hospital. That remarkable record is found in Minneapolis and nowhere else in the world."

Sometimes the difference that orthopedic appliances made was practical. In the days when virtually nothing was accessible, to walk—often with crutches, often in pain and fatigue, often wearing out one's fragile joints—meant that one could gain some limited access: In the 1930s Robert Huse realized that he would have to walk, however "crudely," in order to get an education; if he stayed a wheelchair user he would be shut out of school.

VARIATIONS ON THE THEME
OF VACCINATION

I

The Official Story

In the official stories of the triumph over polio—the ones that appear on the March of Dimes Web site and in books and articles that celebrate the discovery of the Salk vaccine—some combination of the following words appears: "scourge . . . suffering . . . paralysis . . . tragedy . . . odyssey . . . victim . . . pain . . . fear . . . grip . . . severe . . . battle . . . terror . . . tragedy . . . senseless . . . spirit . . . freedom . . . grateful . . . hero . . . triumph . . . monumental . . . historic."

In *A Paralyzing Fear: The Triumph Over Polio in America*:

Those long polio summers tested the American people's will to live, to transcend pain and fear, and to forge their energies in the conquest of a cruel virus. . . . [E]pidemic disease fundamentally changes who we are as a people and how we coalesce to combat an unseen enemy. . . . The victims lived in isolated rural communities, crowded cities, and pristine suburbs. The only thing they had in common was the tragic fact that most were children. . . . But what made it such a vivid terror was the number of paralyzed victims who lived . . . they were a constant reminder of the crippled, breathless aftermath of this most terrible plague. . . . Early experiments led

to tragedy. . . . Some children were paralyzed by the injection. . . . This is
truly an extraordinary triumph.

On the March of Dimes Web site—"50 years of triumph over disease"—the story begins:

> On August 11, 1921, Franklin D. Roosevelt awoke to find that his legs
> were paralyzed. . . . This was the beginning of an historical odyssey for
> both a future U.S. president and a nation in the throes of a mysterious dis-
> ease that devastated untold thousands of children every year. . . . Polio:
> Scourge of Generations . . . a nation gripped by fear. . . . Volunteers Bring
> New Hope to Victims. . . . Victory Close at Hand. . . . [F]reedom for our
> children through the March of Dimes.

II

The Polio Pioneers

Schoolchildren lined up: gap-toothed girls with puff-sleeved dresses and
pigtails; crewcut, towheaded boys who dreamed of becoming cowboys or
firemen. A nurse—dressed as nurses always were in those days, in a white
uniform with a starched cap bobby-pinned to her stiff coiffure—dabbed
their arms with an alcohol-soaked swab. The nurse sings out softly, "Just
a little pinch! There you go! All done!" "Just a little pinch! There you go!
All done!" "Just a little pinch. . . ."

Maybe one girl, having passed through the line, kept mouthing
"Ow-ow-ow!" while she shook her arm up and down. Maybe another
girl proclaimed, in both amazement and pride, "I didn't cry! I didn't cry
at all!"

The kids were all given big black-and-white buttons to pin on their
shirts or dresses that said, "I'm a Polio Pioneer." A newspaper photographer bent down on one knee; his flashbulb went off in a blaze of light. For
the rest of the day the kids were dizzy with excitement: *My picture is going to be in the newspaper! I'm a Polio Pioneer!*

The photographs of those grinning children appeared on the covers of books. Those buttons children were given to wear have become collectibles, are offered for sale on eBay from time to time. The earlier polio pioneers generally get mentioned in the text of books about the race for the vaccine, but there are no glossy pictures of them.

Salk's early tests of his vaccine were carried out at the Polk State School in Pennsylvania, an institution that still described its inhabitants with a term that suggests Victorian sensibilities—the "feeble-minded." Some of the people warehoused there were what we would call intellectually disabled today, although a pictorial history shows a large number of wheelchair users—many inmates may have had cerebral palsy and spina bifida. Nearly all the residents had probably become severely institutionalized, whatever initial impairments they may have had overlaid by the trauma of separation from their families, lack of intellectual stimulation, out-and-out brutality, and the need to fit their psyches and physical needs around the demands of an institution.

A 1946 pamphlet put out by the Pennsylvania Department of Welfare surveyed the twenty-two institutions run by the state and described one of those institutions as having, like any city, "its good and its bad sectors . . . its slums and its Rittenhouse Squares," naming a fashionable area of Philadelphia. The Salk vaccine was tested in the slums of Polk School: One of Salk's assistants felt she would have quit if she'd had to continue visiting the grim back wards for men. The Salk vaccine was also tested at the D. T. Watson Home for Crippled Children, which had been established by the legacy of a prominent Pittsburgh attorney and his wife as "a home for destitute poor white female children between the ages of three and sixteen years, especially including and preferring children crippled or deformed."

Could these back-ward inmates at the Polk School speak, understand language? Probably some of them couldn't. People were often institutionalized shortly after birth, and, like nearly anyone in such circumstances, they would never have learned language, or they had only rudimentary speech. So there was no way to explain to them, as the nurse did to the official Polio Pioneers: "Just a quick pinch. . . . There. . . . All done!" Think of infants getting an injection: the start and wail of pain; the confusion on their faces. And there's no mother to rock them and whisper, "It's all over, sweetie. It's all over." And the vaccine testing didn't involve just a single prick: blood draws were done, too; veins were probed, needles rested inside while blood was drawn out. Strong arms must have had to wrestle the men into compliance, hold them down: Or perhaps restraints were used, patients forced into a wooden chair, leather straps tightened around their limbs.

Salk wasn't the first to test a polio vaccine on institutionalized people. Researchers tested an oral vaccine at Letchworth Village, an institution that had been established in 1907 for the "feeble minded and epileptic" on the west bank of the Hudson River in upstate New York. A rutted dirt road led from there to the New York Reconstruction Home, where those recovering from polio were sent to be "remade" following their encounter with the virus. Leonard Kriegel recalled his visits to Letchworth from the Reconstruction Home:

> Like a tank driver, I maneuvered my chair's bulky presence down the rutted dirt road that led from the hospital to Letchworth Village, a state home for the mentally retarded that we boys, our verbal cruelty as much a mark of our crippled state as our wheelchairs and braces and crutches, derisively called "Crazytown."

Administrators at Letchworth Village worried about the possibility of a polio outbreak among the inmates—not only because epidemics often spread in institutions but because conditions at Letchworth were so hellish that inmates were known to throw feces at one another and also at times to devour their own and that of other inmates—ideal conditions for spreading the virus.

In 1952, when the prominent British medical journal *The Lancet* reviewed the research carried out at Letchworth Village, it pointed out a serious ethical problem—the testing was done on subjects who were referred to as "volunteers," although they had been unable to give their consent and the ethical ramifications had been given scant consideration. The editorial was rather flippant, however, saying, "We might yet read in a scientific journal that an experiment was carried out with twenty volunteer mice." In commenting on this practice John Wilson asked, in *Margin of Safety*—a book about the American "race for the vaccine" from a more detached British perspective:

> Is all human life equally valuable? Christian dogma says it is, but how many of us in our hearts really believe that this is true? If it is absolutely necessary to carry out an experiment, which may possibly be dangerous, is it not rea-

sonable to carry it out on a hopeless imbecile rather than on a normal person? Nobody will officially sanction a policy of this kind, but in fact doctors have been making such selections for years, quietly and without fuss, on occasions when humanity and common sense seemed to demand it.

Wilson, at least, was honest, and willing to speak frankly about a set of ongoing practices and beliefs.

We should remember that the notion of informed consent to medical experiments arose directly from the horror at medical experiments carried out in Nazi concentration camps on those they believed to be subhuman. It makes far more sense to carry out medical experiments on those who can understand not just the procedures being used but the long-range consequences of the experiment. There is rarely a shortage of such volunteers. Thousands upon thousands of people have eagerly taken part in recent trials of experimental AIDS vaccines, with volunteers sometimes actively lobbying the National Institutes of Health to allow clinical trials to proceed. Given how widespread fear of polio was, and how many lives had been touched by the disease, it is hard to believe there wouldn't have been plenty of true volunteers willing to test the polio vaccine.

III

The March of Dimes

There was no end to the hoopla surrounding the fight, the battle, the war, the crusade against the Great Crippler—the search for a vaccine. Every January 30, FDR's birthday, in the good old Mickey-Rooney-Judy-Garland-Let's-Put-on-a-Show! spirit, President's Birthday Balls were held across the country. One year the program for the New York ball, held at the Waldorf, showed a theologically incorrect but nonetheless quite fetching female angel, wearing the American flag as a stole, bending tenderly over a group of blond-haired children. Another year the program featured another angel, carrying a banner that read HEALTH FOR ALL, hovering above another gaggle of sweet-faced white children. Every year Eleanor Roosevelt posed beaming before yet another ornate cake, so large they seemed have come from the hand of an architect rather than a pastry chef. One year the cake looked like the Chrysler Building, another year it resembled the great temple-pyramid at Tikal, Guatemala. And every year there were President's Birthday Ball posters. One shows a soigné couple caught in mid-dip, in full color, while two dark silhouettes gaze up at them. A silhouetted crutch brings home the message: DANCE SO THAT OTHERS MAY WALK.

Comedian and radio star Eddie Cantor went on the air and appealed to the good folks who could hear his voice to send a dime—just one thin dime!—right to the president at the White House to fight this terrible disease. He was riffing on the phrase "March of Time," the name of the newsreels that prefaced almost every movie-house feature. A few days later a mail truck pulled up to the back of the White House with twenty-three bags of mail. It didn't stop there. A day later 150,000 letters were delivered, thirty times the usual number. The White House was so swamped with these dimes it couldn't find official mail. The business of the executive branch nearly ground to a halt. The dimes came in "fixed with gummy tape, baked into cakes, jammed into cans, imbedded in wax and glued into profiles of the President."

Thus was the March of Dimes born. During the forties volunteers passed up and down the aisles of Rialto and Orpheum theaters all across America, jiggling their collection cans. When television came on the scene and Americans shut themselves up inside their homes and stared at their fuzzy black-and-white boxes, the good folks at the National Foundation for Infantile Paralysis renamed the drive the Mothers March. Women went door to door with their collection cans. Sometimes the mothers literally set off marching. One picture shows a regiment of women being led by Ellen Fairclough, Canada's first woman cabinet minister. The regiment's uniforms were sensible cloth coats; and they aren't carrying, of course, rifles and rucksacks, but purses hanging from their left arms, collection cans in their right. One year stage and screen stars Raymond Massey and Tyrone Power joined the fight, wearing placards around their neck reading TONIGHT I AM A MOTHER.

It wasn't just the swells dancing at the Waldorf-Astoria to the tunes played by ten different orchestras; people also danced in places like Weirton, West Virginia, and Clarkston, Michigan. Some balls charged a mere nickel for entry. In one town the door prizes included a bottle of shampoo and a ton of coal. A ball was even held at the Japanese internment camp in Topaz, Utah.

In 1944 FDR likened the war on polio to the wider war being waged:

"Victory is imperative on all fronts. Not until we have removed the shadow of the Crippler from the future of every child can we furl the flags of battle and still the trumpets of attack. The fight against infantile paralysis is a fight to the finish, and the terms are unconditional surrender."

No appeal was too maudlin. On a billboard a child with leg braces seated in a wicker wheelchair warned and pleaded at the same time: "I could be your child." A pouty youngster stared down from a wartime billboard, but the kid had a good reason to pout—poor little thing, in bed with polio. "Please, Mister," she begged passersby, "do your best—and you *can* by making your Donation."

Charity fund-raising invokes fear and pity. Adults and teenagers also got polio, but rarely did charity appeals include the postpubescent. Children tugged at heartstrings in a way that adults did not. America was far more comfortable with the image of the vulnerable child who was already assumed to be in an inferior position. The adult with a disability raised uncomfortable questions about workplace accommodation and sexuality that society preferred to ignore.

Giving became a way of protecting yourself. Go out and ring doorbells for the March of Dimes, and your children will be safe. Eat right and exercise, and you'll stay healthy. Work hard, and you'll get better.

On September 10, 2001, I was in downtown Los Angeles. I passed a down-and-out man on the street who had a dog on a rope leash. The dog skittered backward a bit at my approach, frightened by my power chair, and I held out my hand so it could smell the scent of my dog. "What's your dog's name?" I asked. "Fawn," he said. "You know, like a baby deer." His voice sounded wheezy. I looked up. He had a tracheotomy so he could breathe through his windpipe, like my friend Barbara—who had died a little while before—had had. "I'm trying to get a place to spend the night," he told me. "Do you think you could help me out?" I'd just been to the cash machine. All I had were twenties, and I gave him one.

The next day, September 11, as I rolled through the streets of Los Angeles, not knowing what might happen next, I kept reassuring myself. I gave that man twenty bucks; I'm a good person; nothing bad will happen to me. I knew it was silly and superstitious; I knew it made absolutely no sense; I knew being good or not being good had nothing to do with who lived or died on that day; but still I kept reassuring myself: I gave that man twenty dollars. I will be okay.

Every year the March of Dimes chose its national poster child. One year it was a boy in a Hopalong Cassidy outfit who got lifted onto President Truman's desk. Another year it was a poster baby for whom a photo op was arranged with Santa. For some reason—perhaps the general spirit of overkill—there were six Santas, the sight of whom set the poster baby wailing uncontrollably. Sweet girls in ruffled dresses and metal braces waved to the crowds gathered at the Waldorf. The choice of poster child was announced in the *New York Times*.

Everybody joined the fight. A sideshow midget and giant joined together to collect for the National Foundation, as did Frank Sinatra, Douglas Fairbanks Jr., Grace Kelly, Duke Ellington, Lucille Ball and Desi Arnaz, Marilyn Monroe, Louis Armstrong, Liberace—and don't forget Kokomo Jr., "America's Favorite TV Chimp," who, dressed in a pinstriped suit and a bow tie, held up the banner reading "Join—March of Dimes." America's Sweetheart, the aging Mary Pickford, was shown with a giant top hat in which donations were to be collected. Parades were held along Broadway. In Hartford, Connecticut, they vowed to collect a mile of dimes, and they did it—92,160 dimes. In Times Square a replica of the Trevi Fountain was built—toss a coin over your shoulder just as they do in Rome—toss in your dimes, your quarters, your pennies, your nickels. A helpful sign let visitors know that the Trevi Fountain was in Rome, and that Rome was in Italy.

To some observers of the United States from afar, our "restless belief in the perfectibility of human affairs," our having "discarded resignation as a virtue," and our "constant striving for improvement," always endemic, became, during our dash for the vaccine against polio, epidemic.

The notion of "racing for the cure" has become so deeply entrenched that there are any number of literal races—on bike and foot—to raise money for the cure for AIDS, breast cancer, and multiple sclerosis. "Race for the Cure" is now a registered trademark of the Susan G. Komen Breast Cancer Foundation, and a vice president for the PR firm for the corporate sponsor of the Tanqueray AIDS Ride spoke of the AIDS ride as having achieved "brand equity."

IV

The Father of Vaccination

Just as a murkier history is revealed as the usual history of the polio pioneers is peeled away, a similar story lies behind the creation of vaccination itself. Edward Jenner, an eighteenth-century British physician, is generally credited with the invention of the technique itself. Jenner learned the country wisdom that someone infected with cowpox—a mild disease contracted from cows—was thereafter immune from smallpox. In 1796 he took pus from cowpox lesions on the hand of a young dairymaid, Sarah Nelmes. Shortly thereafter he inoculated an eight-year-old boy, James Phipps, his gardener's son, who developed a fever but had none of the other symptoms of cowpox. Six weeks later he inoculated James with smallpox matter and found that he was immune to infection. History has not recorded how James Phipps or his parents felt about his initial inoculation with cowpox or his subsequent exposure to sometimes fatal smallpox. After doing more experiments—including one on his own eleven-month-old son—Jenner published his monograph, *An Inquiry into the Causes and Effects of the Variolae Vaccinae,* whose prose style stands in such contrast to our current medical writing that I can't resist quoting from its opening sentences, which preface his discussion of cowpox:

> The deviation of man from the state in which he was originally placed by nature seems to have proved to him a prolific source of diseases. From the love of splendour, from the indulgences of luxury, and from his fondness for amusement he has familiarised himself with a great number of animals, which may not originally have been intended for his associates.

> The wolf, disarmed of ferocity, is now pillowed in the lady's lap. The cat, the little tiger of our island, whose natural home is the forest, is equally domesticated and caressed. The cow, the hog, the sheep, and the horse, are all, for a variety of purposes, brought under his care and dominion.

That Jenner is credited as the inventor of vaccination seems strange, since what he did seems little more than a refinement of practices that had been used for millennia. Inoculation—deliberate, immunity-providing infection with a very small amount of infected pus or other matter from someone with a mild case of a disease—had been practiced since 1000 B.C. in China and India. When Lady Mary Wortley Montagu was in Constantinople with her husband, the British ambassador, she learned of the practice. In 1717 she wrote to a friend, "The smallpox, so fatal and so general amongst us, is here entirely harmless by the invention of engrafting (which is the term they give it)." Montagu wrote about attending a party held for this purpose. An old woman entered with a nutshell full of "matter of the best sort of smallpox" and went around opening veins on the guests' arms with a needle. Montagu, whose face was permanently scarred as a result of a girlhood bout with smallpox, determined to bring this method to England, although she feared that physicians there would not have "virtue enough to destroy such a considerable branch of their revenue for the good of mankind."

On her return to England Montagu persuaded Caroline, Princess of Wales, to inoculate two of her daughters, although the method was first tried on six condemned criminals—who were rewarded with their freedom—and a number of hapless orphans.

V

Polio Vaccine and Aids

In the science section of the *New York Times,* I read an article about a book that posits the theory that HIV came from SIV (simian immunodeficiency virus), not, as many suspect, as a result of simians biting humans or humans preparing and eating monkey meat but rather from chimpanzee kidney tissue allegedly being used in the preparation of an experimental oral polio vaccine—the one developed under the leadership of Hilary Koprowski, who administered a version of it to the inmates at Letchworth Village in upstate New York. The most graphic evidence of the theory is a map that claims to show the places where the suspect pool of vaccine was given, and early outbreaks of the HIV virus. The purported correlation is eerie. Koprowski, with the support of many scientists and doctors, has vigorously denied the allegations.

When I spot the book—called *The River: A Journey to the Source of*

HIV and AIDS—on the shelf at the library, I'm amazed at the thickness of it—it's more than a thousand pages. (The last two-hundred-odd pages are devoted to notes, citing articles with names like "Population Genetic Studies in the Congo. I. Glucose-6-Phosphate Dehydrogenase Deficiency, Hemoglobin S and Malaria" and "Immunization of Children by the Feeding of Living Attenuated Type 1 and Type 2 Poliomyelitis Virus and the Intramuscular Injection of Immune Serum Globulin.") I'd expected a slim volume—after all, how much evidence could there be to muster? It's not just long, I discover when I get it home, but dense. I'm a fast reader, but this book takes me nearly a week to work through.

Until I read this book I'd never understood how people could get engaged in the long-winded reality of live trials broadcast on Court TV. I preferred the tautness of a good detective story.

But reading Edward Hooper's monumental work, I understood that this was a different kind of detective story. In the fictionalized detective story, there is always an essential fact that makes the story come to a climax: The purloined letter is right there, all along, on the mantel; the casing of the Maltese Falcon is chipped away to reveal plaster of Paris. Facts are in short supply. But in this case it is just the opposite: There is an abundance of facts, a cornucopia of them, a plethora, more facts than you know what to do with. Figuring out what to ignore is crucial.

I let the dishes pile up in the sink so I could read the book; I took the dog on abbreviated walks. One morning I woke up with tendinitis flaring in my wrists, and I realized I'd been stressing my hands by holding this massive book.

It is chilling to read about the slipshod way vaccines were tested on African people. If what Hooper reports is true, they were treated more haphazardly than guinea pigs in laboratories, which, after all, are kept track of, assigned identification numbers, have records kept about them. Between February and April 1958, an international team of vaccinators traveled through what was then the Belgian Congo, squirting vaccine into the mouths of some 215,504 people—the vaccinators kept track of the number of doses given but not to whom they were given. A photograph from that campaign shows a white woman in a pith helmet giving vaccine to a baby in the foreground, while in the distance what was described as a "sea of Africans" stretches to the edge of the frame.

In 1963 J. R. Wilson wrote in *Margin of Error:* "The measures designed to protect the world from polio may, in their turn, for all we know, lead to some other quite unexpected consequence which may be to man's disadvantage."

If you accept even the possibility that Hooper's thesis is correct (and many scientists don't), those words have a chillingly prophetic ring to them.

VI

The End?

The campaign for the global eradication of polio has been stymied by fears that the polio vaccine is part of a Western plot to sterilize African women. Press reports of this usually hint at African and/or Muslim irrationality, the quixotic beliefs of Muslim clerics in "plots" fomented by Westerners. This boycott has its point of origin in Kano, in northern Nigeria, where Pfizer carried out a controversial 1996 drug study in which an experimental antibiotic was tested on children with meningitis. Because the experimental antibiotic may have been less effective than other drugs, it has been alleged that the meningitis caused the deaths of several children and left others with disabilities. Some parents contend they were unaware their children were taking part in an experiment, and the fear that African children are again being used as unwitting experimental subjects has fueled the boycott of the polio vaccine. Pfizer has denied any wrongdoing and says that it received consent from the families.

Even in the broader public health community, the drive to eradicate polio is controversial, with arguments made that resources could be more usefully spent on diseases that are more prevalent and cause far more deaths, such as malaria and tuberculosis. Are the needs of donors to feel good about the final eradication of a disease being given more weight than the needs of the countries receiving aid? Is the eradication of polio a victory that could be achieved, partially eclipsing the wider failures—not just in the continued global devastation of AIDS, but in the ongoing deaths of children in the third world, more than 10 million of whom, according to UNICEF, die every year from such preventable causes as malnutrition and contaminated water?

THERAPY

The women rub their hands together to warm them.

They touch me: my ankles, the bottoms of my feet, my knees. My shoulders, my arms, my neck.

Parts of my body are tender: I warn them to be careful.

They used to urge me on: "Just one more. Great. How about *one* more." Now—when the medical profession has realized that rehabilitation can have a downside, triggering or worsening postpolio syndrome, they warn me to stop before I get tired, not to push myself.

Every week my mother drove me from our house in Hamilton to the hospital in Utica for physical therapy. Sometimes my baby brother was in the "way back" of the station wagon, sleeping on a blanket laid across the wicker laundry basket, atop a pile of clothes waiting to be ironed. Sometimes my mother had to put her foot on the brake and stop the car and wait while a farmer urged his herd of Holsteins across the road, moving them from the milking barn to the pasture. Having just been milked, their flat udders, the long teats distended, swung from side to side.

From watching my mother while she drove, I had figured out that the car went forward when the pedal closer to me was pushed and stopped when the pedal farther away was pushed. I bragged to my sisters that I knew how to *drive*. Staring out the window as my mother and I made our weekly trek to Utica, passing the marshes with the redwing blackbirds rising from them, the patchwork quilt of fields, I imagined President Eisenhower passing a special law that would allow me, Anne Finger, of Hamilton, New York, to get a license at the age of five, since I had figured out driving all by myself.

The odor of warm chlorine rose from the pool, filling the blue-tiled room. My mother lifted me onto the padded table covered in brown leather and unbuckled the leather straps of my braces, tugging my legs free from them, my feet free from the square orthopedic shoes. Dressed in my bathing suit, I was lowered into the outstretched arms of a physical therapist and from there into the pool. My mother sat in a corner waiting for me. Do I remember her reading while she waited for me? No, but she must have. Maybe Carson McCullers's *The Ballad of the Sad Café* or James Baldwin's *Go Tell It on the Mountain,* in paperback, or a hardcover she had checked out from the library. Or maybe she held my brother in her arms, although she may have left him sleeping in the car—ordinary parenting then, not considered neglect—going out to check on him every now and again.

Our voices echoed off the tile walls, off the water. The sloshing sounds we made as we moved through the water echoed faintly, too. A continuous minor vibrato shadowed our speech, our movements. The reflections of the harsh fluorescent lights above were broken up and refracted in the water. Steam dripped down the distant windows, panes of milky glass with what looked like chicken wire sandwiched between them. The edges of the pool were sharp, as was the noise of the weights clanking against one another as they were lifted up and down in the therapy room next door, and the squeaks of gurney wheels rolling by. Everything was simultaneously muffled and distinct: as if Monet's garden at Giverny had been painted by a hyperrealist.

Decades later, when I saw the film *Coming Home,* with one of its opening scenes set in a VA rehab hospital, wounded Vietnam vets undergoing therapy in a pool, I heard those particular sounds again—the sloshing of water, the echoes of the sloshing of water—and felt a sense of familiarity and shock as one of my most intimate moments reverberated through the crowded theater.

The physical therapists, who of course were women, wore one-piece blue bathing suits, sometimes navy, sometimes robin's egg, and off-white bathing caps with straps that snapped under their chins. The women all had short hair, permanent-waved into tight curls. After they pulled the bathing caps over their heads, they worked their hands along the joining of cap and head, shoving errant locks of hair under them.

It was important for women to keep their hair dry in those days. It didn't matter for men, since they all had crewcuts. If a woman's hair got wet, her hairdo would be ruined. "I just washed my hair," women used to say, "and I can't do a thing with it." One time, at my aunt Dorothy's house, we were watching a quiz show—*To Tell the Truth* or *What's My Line?*—and Kitty Carlisle or Dorothy Kilgallen was wearing a turban. A turban seemed the height of New York City glamour. But then my aunt pronounced, "I guess *she* just washed her hair."

Advertisements asked, "Which Twin Has the Toni?" and showed identical twins with identical hairstyles—one had been done at a beauty parlor at the astronomical cost of fifteen dollars and the other had been done with the economical Toni Home Permanent Wave.

I had a permanent once. My mother sat me on the top step of the blue wooden stool, with my head stretched backward over the kitchen sink. She dabbed my hair, wrapped up in pink plastic rollers with the chemical that was described in the handy instruction booklet as the "developer," a perfumed concoction made primarily of ammonia. The fumes were so strong I tasted them, chemical and sharp, in the back of my throat, reminding me instantly of the taste of ether. As the ammonia fumes licked the back of my mouth, I squirmed and hollered, "It's in my throat! It's in my throat!" My mother told me to cut it out, adding: "You have to suffer to be beautiful." Even then I knew she did not mean this. She believed some things were worth suffering for, but beauty was not one of them. After all that my hair stayed curly for only a day before it flopped straight again. And even during that single day when my face was wreathed by curls, I did not look beautiful, as I had expected. The inability of my hair to curl seemed part and parcel of my square orthopedic shoes, of my clanking metal braces with their leather straps and pads that smelled of old sweat and saddle soap.

When I was four or five, my hair was cut in bangs and chopped off just below my ears. Did I wear a bathing cap when I went into the therapy pool? I must have. Wet hair was thought to cause colds.

In the pool I could do all kinds of things I could not do on land. I could lift my right leg straight up, over and over again. I could move it out to the side and back and lift it up behind me. Every week we repeated these motions over and over again, pretending that this was somehow going to translate into making me stronger on dry land. But it didn't.

Every night, after the dinner dishes had been washed, I would lie on the kitchen table, and my mother and I would do my exercises. Sit-ups to strengthen my abdominal muscles. Scissoring my legs open and then closed, my mother helping to move my right leg. Leg lifts—again with my mother providing all but a fraction of the movement for my right leg. "Passive" exercise, where my mother moved a part of my right leg that had no muscle strength at all.

We were patient. We were working hard. We did not give up. Results were bound to come. We must not become discouraged. The God we didn't believe in was a God who helped those who helped themselves.

Sometimes my therapy wasn't given in the pool but in the physical therapy gym. Blue mats spread on the floor. Green parallel bars, which I used to practice walking, looking as if they had been made from plumbing pipe. Various tables, padded in brown leather, on which I lay while the therapists repeated the exercises I did on the kitchen table each night after dinner. Plaques and posters with inspirational sayings: "The only place where success comes before hard work is in the dictionary." A drawing of the tortoise crossing the finish line before the hare. "Slow and steady wins every time." A drawing of a ladder, on whose bottom rung were the words "I can't do it," followed by "I might try, but just once." "I am trying to do it, but it hurts," and finally ending with "I did it!"

My therapy, at least, was never painful.

A man in his sixties, who underwent postpolio rehabilitation at the Sister Kenny Institute as a boy, remembered male physical therapists—he described them as gorillas—who forced his body to bend forward while he screamed in pain. As we talked on the phone, his voice caught, choked. "Are you crying?" I asked. My own eyes were filling with tears.

"Yes," he said. He sounded embarrassed, sobbing over the phone to a stranger. He apologized.

"It's all right," I murmured.

"I'm sorry," he said.

"Really, it's all right."

"It was—it was tough."

Certainly it makes sense to ease muscle contractures, permanent short-ening of the muscles, since they can cause pain and restricted range of motion. When I was in Bombay at the World Social Forum—an interna-tional gathering of antiglobalization activists—in January 2004, I met two disabled men who shared a single wheelchair, one sitting on the seat, the other on the footrests, who had journeyed to the forum from Ra-jasthan, in India's north. "Handicaps helping handicaps," one of them said, explaining their arrangement. After so much time spent with dis-abled people, I am pretty good at guessing people's impairments: I was quite sure the man who sat on the footrests had had polio. His arms and legs were frozen, nearly immobile. This man would have benefited from physical therapy—but it could have been gentle and slow stretching, not the brutal wrenching we so often experienced.

In some corner of my brain I believed that lie, that with enough grit and determination and hard work we could do anything. My mother read *The Little Engine That Could* over and over again. "I think I can. I think I can." I don't believe in burning books, but I could make an exception for *The Little Engine That Could*. That lie we were fed, that determination would conquer all. The psychic damage it caused.

I knew that my disability would never completely go away, but for more decades than I care to remember, in some corner of my brain I believed—despite the daily evidence otherwise—that I would someday be-come a woman with a slight, stiff-legged limp. I believed this despite the fact I have only one functioning muscle in my right leg—a quadriceps I variously describe as "pathetic" or "like a strand of overcooked vermi-celli." In order to walk I must tilt my entire body to the left, hitch up my right side, and, using my abdominal muscles and the muscles of my but-tocks, fling my right leg forward. Then, in order to transfer weight from my left leg to my right, I have to press my right hand down on my right quadriceps, my hand supplying the force missing from that muscle.

Until I was thirty I believed that if I just tried harder I would get better. I believed this during the time I was swimming a mile a day, and I was not getting any better. Perhaps I just needed to swim two miles, or three. Or five. I believed this during the periods of time when I forced myself to go on long walks of three, four, sometimes five miles. Perhaps I just wasn't walking far enough. No matter how hard I tried, I believed I just wasn't trying hard enough.

One of the myths of polio was the belief that, with enough hard work, recovery would be ongoing. In fact, although muscular function often did return within the first months or even year of illness, there was almost no chance after that of meaningful changes in overall recovery of compromised muscles. Sometimes recovery in those initial months could be rapid and almost astonishing. Some children who had been initially unable to walk might literally be running a few months after the acute phase of the illness ended. Some. Not all. And yet parents were led to believe—and allowed themselves to be led to believe—that progress would continue.

In *No Time for Tears,* Charles H. Andrews wrote:

> It is true that polio remains one of the few diseases known to man for which there is no positive cure—yet.
>
> But we have seen, in the physiotherapy department, a twelve-year-old girl, crippled and twisted from the hips down, learn to walk again. By the time she is in college or is married you will never know that she had polio.
>
> There is a seven-year-old boy in the pool. Three months ago, his parents moved here from another city. He'd been paralyzed for several years. His legs were "frozen" in a cross-legged sitting position. He had to be carried wherever he went. And they said he would never walk again.
>
> Now, with modern physiotherapy techniques, this lad is swimming! Those legs? They are straightened out in the water, moving. Before long he, too, will walk.

My friend Karen, who also had polio, and I laugh, recalling the underarms of our winter coats when we lived on the East Coast and walked on crutches. We would work so hard, walking, working up such a sweat that the underarms of our winter coats would get soaked with perspiration, rings of yellowed stains, like the growth rings in a sawed-off tree trunk.

Leonard Kriegel walked "mile after mile on my braces and crutches. I did hundreds of push-ups every day to build up my arms, shoulders, and chest." After lifting himself repeatedly on the monkey bars in a nearby park, he would return home, working himself "to the point of collapse."

When I was twelve or thirteen I finally got the long leg brace taken off my right leg. It had stretched up my entire leg, with a leather strap—a pelvic band—wrapping around my waist. In order to walk without my brace, I had to press my hand against my right quadriceps. In Guatemala I have seen nondisabled men doing this, men who themselves must weigh far less than fifty kilos, carrying a fifty-kilo sack on their backs secured with a tumpline, struggling up a hill, pushing with their hands to help their legs.

Whenever my father saw me doing this, he told me to stop. He didn't ask me why I was doing it or what would happen if I didn't do it—I would be able to walk only two or three very short steps before my quad got so fatigued it gave out. He said, "Stop doing that with your hand!" the way he would have told me to stop picking my nose.

When my father was in his late seventies he was still downhill skiing, despite asthma and emphysema, huffing and wheezing on the slopes. When the waitress at Friendly's or the Newport Creamery would come to our table and say, "How are you folks doing today?" with her pencil poised above her order pad, my dad would answer: "I've just been skiing. . . . Guess how much I pay for my lift ticket?"

"How much, sir?" she would dutifully ask.

"Five dollars, because I'm over seventy-five. . . . In two years, it'll be free, because I'll be eighty."

I said to people, "He'll probably have a heart attack on the slopes. That's the way he'd like to go."

When he was in his mid-seventies he bought a new hot-water heater for the apartment on the second floor of the coach house behind our house in Providence. He decided he could move the 130-pound hot-water heater up the stairs himself—even though he weighed only a little more than the hot-water heater—by rocking it up the stairs. He got it all the way to the top when he discovered that the door to the apartment was closed. He—and the hot-water heater—tumbled down the stairs together. When I saw him a few weeks later, he had a couple of sores on his nose, and I asked him if they were from his glasses not fitting right across the bridge of his nose. It was then I heard the story of the hot-water heater. When I told him to be more careful, he snapped back, "I'm not just going to sit around and get old."

Did I get my take-no-prisoners!-never-say-die!-full-speed-ahead!-quitters-never-win! attitude from him? Or was it something he absorbed from those years of watching me go through physical therapy, of being told, "She can do it if she sets her mind to it"? Or did I get it from him? Or did we pass it back and forth, him to me, me to him, its force growing synergistically as we exchanged it?

When I was in my mid-forties, and postpolio syndrome had arrived with a wallop, I sat in the office of a doctor who said, "Your nerves are not under your voluntary control. You cannot will them back." I was crying. She put her hand on my shoulder, made eye contact with me, brought her face closer to mine, and said it again. "Your nerves are not under your voluntary control. You cannot will them back."

A few years after that another doctor said, "It's really a miracle that you can walk at all with what you've got." My right leg is a collection of muscles that rate "zero" or "trace" on a manual muscle test. My quadriceps rises, on a good day, to a "one," which means that, when seated, I can use it to lift my right leg upward very slowly three or—on a very good day—four inches above the seat of the chair. I can repeat this action two or three times before becoming exhausted.

It was not true that I could do anything. I knew it, my mother knew it, the physical therapists knew it, the doctors knew it. The neural connections between my brain and many of my muscles were gone. Even if they could have been restored, my muscles had long since atrophied. Nothing would bring them back. I could try—I did try—for years and years and years, and nothing much changed. I hated being told to try. I had tried and tried and tried and tried and tried and tried and tried.

And I didn't particularly want my body to change. I had no memory of not being disabled. My disability was like my femaleness, part of who I was. I had a child's adaptability. My way of doing things may have seemed odd and awkward to other people, but it was my way of doing things. When I blew out the candles on my birthday cakes, I didn't wish to be nondisabled. I wanted a pony, a toy gun, a canopy bed. It was everyone else who wanted this so much for me, who was let down by my not getting better.

Still my mother drove me, every week, between our house in Hamilton and Children's Hospital in Utica. Sometimes we sang together a song from the early days of the Erie Canal: "I've got a mule, her name is Sal/Fifteen miles on the Erie Canal." My mother told me about the early-nineteenth-century barges that had traveled the canals linking—via the Hudson River—the Atlantic Ocean and the Great Lakes. They had been pulled by mules, treading along paths lining the canals. The bridges over the canal were so low that when one was approached someone would call out, "Low bridge! Everybody down!" and the bargemen would scramble to lie facedown on the deck.

One day on the way home, my mother took me on a side trip to see the Nine Mile Swamp, which the Loomis Gang, a nineteenth-century troop of horse thieves and scoundrels, had used as their base. Were there kids with the surname of Loomis at Hamilton Central? There may have been. The name is a common one in that part of upstate New York. It was Ezra Pound's original middle name, after his grandmother, who had come from nearby Oneida County. He changed it to "Weston" on arriving at Hamilton College in Clinton, New York, not wanting to be associated with the gang whose exploits were still fresh in local memory.

My mother parked the car on a rutted road with grass growing down the center where it hadn't been tamped down by car tires. Ghostlike gray trunks of dead trees rose out of the boggy water. The marsh smelled fetid. A bird called from deep in the woods. I wanted to leave. Was it because I was frightened? Or because I was disappointed?

Disappointed, I think. When we were eight years old, Debby and I used to watch a Disney series called *The Swamp Fox. The Swamp Fox*—based on a true story!—was about a Revolutionary general, Francis Marion, who waged a guerrilla campaign from the swamps of South Carolina. Saturday afternoons, Debbie and I would watch it on the black-and-white television in her den, our fascination with the series made all the sharper by our knowledge that, unlike *The Lone Ranger* or *Sky King*, it would end at a definite date.

I was old enough to know that television was make-believe, but young enough that when I saw a portrait of the real Francis Marion—I must have looked him up in the encyclopedia at the library—I was acutely disappointed. He was fine featured, with bulging eyes and a priggish cast to his mouth. He looked nothing like the actor who played him on television—the handsome and dashing Leslie Nielsen, not yet the amiable buffoon of *Airplane!* and *Surf Ninjas* movies. At Nine Mile Swamp I had half expected to be transported back in time, to see the flash of a horse's tail disappearing into the marsh, perhaps even fantasized about Leslie Nielsen swooping down to carry me off with him to fight the British.

On one of the routes—my mother varied them because she got bored driving the same roads, there and back, week after week—we passed a garage that had a tin sign with the Michelin tire man on it. Only years later did I realize that he was supposed to look as if he were made from tires. At the time his strange protrusions of flesh just seemed grotesque; his smile and raised hand malevolent, as if he were about to tear himself free from the sign and come after me. I'd turn my head away when I knew we were getting close to him. But then, at the last minute, I'd have to look, just to make sure he wasn't escaping from the sign to chase us. Or maybe I looked hoping that the sign had been taken down. As soon as I looked, I'd regret it. There he was again, bloblike, his image made fresh again so he could haunt me when I lay down in bed that night.

Sometimes we went a different route, longer but special, because we got to go by the billboard for Dutch Boy paints, with its working teeter-totter, rocking back and forth, the Dutch boy on one side, the Dutch girl on the other—both, of course, wearing wooden shoes. My mother used to go by that sign when she drove to Syracuse to see me in the hospital there, and I would often ask her when she arrived for visiting hours if the Dutch boy and Dutch girl were still going up and down.

Most days we went on no side excursions. I loved to stare at the broken lines on the highway, the way they seemed to disappear as we drove over them, or to tilt my head back so that the world was skewed and the blur of trees, punctuated by telephone poles, seemed a work of abstract art. Occasionally we'd see the carcasses of woodchucks, cats, even a deer, squashed by the of the road, or smell the rank odor of a dead skunk.

We drove past bleak nineteenth-century mills, long since abandoned. Much of the land we drove across belonged to the Oneida Nation, but it wasn't until decades later, after a decision by the U.S. Supreme Court, that the Oneida would make a move to enforce their ownership. When we lived there, the only evidence of the once-powerful Iroquois Confederacy were the names of places—Oneida, Seneca Falls, Mohawk, Chenango, Chittenango Falls, Oneonta, Skaneateles, Schenectady—and the names of products—Iroquois Indian Head Beer, Mohawk Gasoline.

Decades later our roles are reversed, and I am the one taking my mother for medical treatment, twice a day driving her from her house in Pawtucket to Rhode Island Hospital. She sits in the passenger seat, and I am behind the wheel of a rental car equipped with hand controls. From her seat my mother keeps the world in line, offering reproving comments as we drive through the Providence streets: to fleshy women in skimpy tops ("Oh, dear—you are just too big to be wearing that!"; to immigrant shopkeepers who have posted signs on which they betray their naive belief that the English language follows logical spelling rules; drivers of gas guzzlers ("Don't they understand about global warming?"); drivers of cars that fail to come to a complete stop at stop signs ("Stop means stop!"); drivers of cars with windows rolled down blasting rap music; and most grievous of all, of course, gas guzzlers thumping rap music *and* rolling through stop signs. Of course none of the offenders hear these comments. Only I do. It seems important to her that I know these affronts are not passing unnoticed.

Did she issue similar reprimands to the world when she and I drove between Hamilton and Utica? I don't think so. The upstate New York world of that time was more in synch with her ideas of what should and should not be. Although I remember once seeing a sign in Utica that said "BBQ" and asking her what it meant, and the sharpness of her answer. She let me know not only that it stood for "barbecue" but also that this was not a proper abbreviation—akin to the horrors of "Xmas" and "Thruway." There was also something "seedy"—most likely the word she would have used, had she been forced to use an actual word and not just to indicate her disapproval via tone of voice—about a place with a sign in front that said "BBQ."

I hated hearing about Wilma Rudolph, who had won three gold medals in track in the 1956 Olympics. The tag line about Wilma Rudolph was "A Negro girl from the South who overcame a childhood bout with polio that left her unable to walk for two years, and who went on to win . . ."

Whenever I heard that, I felt a sense of shame. If she could do it, why couldn't I? I also wonder if Rudolph's polio wasn't a legend, a story repeated so often that it took on a life of its own. She may have had polio, but a bout of polio that left one unable to walk for two years could not have receded so completely that she could go on to become a champion runner. Or she may well have had some other ailment—perhaps rheumatoid arthritis, perhaps Guillain-Barré syndrome, perhaps one of the family of Coxsackie viruses that can mimic polio—that was misdiagnosed. Perhaps the misdiagnosis came about through a genuine medical error or perhaps, as sometimes happened, it was done deliberately so that a patient could get the financial assistance given to those with this emblematic disease, funding lacking for other, less famous illnesses. Usually what was diagnosed as polio was the clinical entity "polio," but not always. A recent article in the *Journal of Medical Biography* makes a persuasive case that polio's most famous exemplar, Franklin Delano Roosevelt, was not disabled by polio but by Guillain-Barré syndrome.

And I hated *Heidi*. I felt an acute sense of shame whenever I heard the name, for I would immediately think of the scene in which Heidi's crippled friend, Clara, having had her wheelchair pushed down the mountain by jealous Peter, discovers that she can, after all, walk. It was so easy—all she needed was a bit of encouragement from Heidi: " 'Do it once more,' Heidi urged eagerly." A gingerly step, and a less gingerly step, and soon Clara is traipsing toward the alpine meadow.

Now I find in *Heidi* disturbing presentiments of the Nazi obsessions with health and the *Volk*—and their genocide of disabled people. The German-speaking Heidi, daughter of the soil and the healthy mountain air, is sent to the stone-walled Sesemann house in cosmopolitan Frankfurt to act as companion to sickly Clara. There, deprived of her connection to the earth, breathing the enervating air, rosy-cheeked Heidi comes close to becoming an invalid herself. Health returns only when Heidi and Clara escape the sickening cosmopolitan air and go to the countryside. Sunshine, goat's milk, the spicy smell of new-mown hay, the patchwork quilt of blue gentians and buttercups flung on the mountainside, and soon Clara will undergo her resurrection, rising from her invalid death-in-life to take her rightful place in the alpine pasture, as the wild yellow roses and red centauries, buffeted by the wind, nod their approval. I can almost imagine a troop of Hitler Youth, in lederhosen and swastika armbands, appearing on the crest of a hill, whistling the "Horst Wessel Song" as Clara takes her first tentative steps.

Those years of physical therapy, of being told over and over again, "You can do anything you set your mind to," "Don't give up," "Keep trying," "Work through the pain," had a lifetime effect on nearly everyone I know who has had polio. Since I was such a young child when I had polio and underwent rehabilitation, when my character was still being formed, those messages became part of the core of who I am. When I was in my forties, driving from Detroit to an artists' colony in the Pacific Northwest, I called my sister Jane in Seattle in the early evening, from a phone booth in Missoula, Montana, and said, "I'm going to try to get to your place tonight."

"You'll never make it."

I laughed. "You never should have said that. Now I'm going to drive all night if I have to." I had the ability to laugh with ironic detachment at my obsessions, at my I'll-prove-to-you-I-can-do-it, but still they remained. I got back in my Volvo and I drove. I drove and I drove and I drove and I drove. *I think I can, I think I can, I think I can.* Did I fall asleep while driving that night? I don't remember, although I have done so many times—what finally broke me of the habit was waking up as my car was veering off the highway.

I didn't make it from Missoula to Seattle that night, giving up around two or three in the morning in the Utah panhandle. The next morning I got in the car and started driving again. My neck and my shoulders and my left leg were aching, and I pulled off the highway and stopped at a Kmart or a SavMor pharmacy to buy the house brand of Tylenol. I decided it would be stupid to drive around this town looking for a place where I could get a skim milk latte, so I decided to go instead to the drive-up window of a Burger King and tell the squawky box I wanted a large coffee with two creams and four sugars. But somehow I didn't find a Burger King—instead, I found myself back on the highway, coffeeless, with nothing to wash down my Knol or nonaspirin pain reliever.

I got off the highway five (yes, five) more times that morning, each time intending to take the house brand of Tylenol, and each time somehow managing to forget and found myself back on the highway, driving too fast along the interstate, with my neck and shoulders hurting so much I couldn't think about anything else but how much pain I was in.

And then, finally having swallowed the Tylenol, I drove down out of the Rockies and across the Columbia River Gorge. I feel a physical love for the West—perhaps "lust" would be a better term—for the vastness of that landscape, for its emptiness and wildness. There have been few times in my life when happiness has hit me with the force of a blow: One of them was the day in 1976 when I was headed to California for the first time, in my blue Ford Pinto; leaving behind the cornfields of Iowa (corn, corn, and more corn, who could possibly eat all that corn?), the drear of the Nebraska prairie, my overloaded Pinto struggling slowly up the grade into the Rockies, and then the vast sky opening up above me, the sight of thunderstorms in the far distance, the beauty of that crippled landscape.

This part of the drive is almost as beautiful. Why had I been pushing myself to drive across it in the dark? Just because my sister had said, "You'll never make it," and something in me wanted to prove her wrong?

On the way back from the hospital, my mother would buy me a nickel box of Cracker Jack in the red-and-white box with the picture of a sailor, a cap set on his head, saluting and winking. I'd always open my box of Cracker Jack from the bottom, hoping to retrieve the prize sooner. From time to time I've bought a box as an adult, but now I'm always disappointed in the chintzy prizes—stickers, a thin plastic figurine. In the 1950s the prizes were miniature books, die-cast metal animals, a magnifying glass through which I studied the whorls of my fingerprints.

We passed gently rolling hillocks called moraines, formed, my mother told me, by ancient glaciers. Sometimes, when we drove by barns, my mother said, "Oh, what a beautiful barn!"

When my son and I were living in Michigan, driving through the countryside beyond Detroit, we would pass a barn, a simple red shape in the middle of a flat and empty field, and I heard myself say, "Oh, what a beautiful barn!" I loved the texture of their wood, battered by wind and rain and time, the simplicity of their forms. Architectural modernism was born here, created by these untutored farmers. And then I told Max, "When I was your age, my mother—your grandmother—used to love barns, and I never understood why. But now I get it. . . . Someday," I said, "maybe you'll have a kid, and you'll love barns, and your kid will think you're a crackpot. Sweetie," I added, but he was giving me his *Yeah-right-ma* look.

HOMESICKNESS

It was March. Beneath the windows of Utica Children's Hospital the snow, accumulating since November, was beginning to melt, the winter's history revealing itself layer by layer, as the ancient cities of Troy, one built atop another, did to Schliemann. The melted snow, along with the automobile exhaust and grime it held, accumulated in brackish puddles, half freezing to slush. At some point there would be a cold snap, and everything would freeze again, the melted water becoming smooth and treacherous ice. If I was walking along the sidewalk then, some grown-up would see me and call out, "Be careful! It's icy!" which I would find amusing and annoying. Of course I knew it was icy. I was as aware of where I set my feet as a mountain climber making an ascent up a sheer rock face. I always walked with my head down, eyeing potential hazards—slate sidewalks, mud, unevenness.

Soon it would be April, and my mother would say, "April is the cruellest month," and, "Whanne that Aprille with his shoures sote . . . ," Even my mother, who could find delight in so many things—the looping shape of the nest the Baltimore oriole built in one of our six maples, the snowdrops and crocuses that would soon push their way up through the sodden ground—could find nothing delightful in this bleak season.

I knew the sound that my rubber boots made, wading through the slush. I remembered, from last March and the Marches before, how the sodden dirty water would find its way down inside my rubber galoshes, dirtying my white ankle socks and the turned-up cuffs of the blue jeans I wore after school and on weekends. I could imagine partially refrozen puddles, topped by a thin glaze of ice; could see myself tapping them with the tip of my crutch and watching the cracks skitter outward.

A civil defense drill was being held. The entire city was supposed to pretend that an atomic bomb was about to explode on top of us. At four o'clock in the afternoon, the air-raid warning sirens went off, and then everyone sheltered indoors for an hour. We were used to this sort of thing. In every public building signs with a black circle with three yellow triangles inside pointed toward the building's fallout shelter. At school we'd been shown a cartoon in which Bert the Turtle pulled into his shell, while a catchy jingle played in the background, telling us to "duck and cover." The year before, during a drill, our third-grade class had gone into the hallway and sat down on the floor, bending our heads down and covering them with our arms. A photographer from the *Mid-York Weekly* took our picture. I had flung my crutches down on the floor, and the photograph of us ran on the front page of the paper, with a caption reading: "A pair of crutches provides a grim reminder of what might happen in the event of atomic war."

During one of my hospital stays my roommate declared to a nurse that she hated another patient—only to be reprimanded: "The Bible tells us not to hate anyone." "But what about Russians?" my roommate asked. "Oh, that's different," the nurse allowed.

At four o'clock we heard the sirens wail. An eerie silence began, the usual ambient noise of cars and horns gone. I turned my head and looked out the window at the empty street that ran alongside the hospital. The entire city was, for an hour at least, as locked down as we were. In far-off New York City, pacifists refused to take part in this drill, courting arrest. The male demonstrators wore suits and white shirts and ties beneath their overcoats, while the women's nylon-clad legs, unprotected by their winter coats, shivered in the cold. In Utica, and in the towns around it—the ones named by homesick white settlers—Paris, Rome, Hanover, as well as the ones with down-to-earth names like Hitching Corner, Irish Settlement, and New York Mills—no one defied the orders given from on high. My parents might have sent, when they could manage it, a check to the National Committee for a SANE Nuclear Policy, or to Martin Luther King's SCLC, but they followed the rules. Although they refused to build a fallout shelter, despite the booklets we brought home from school, with their line drawings showing an aproned Mom, a chisel-jawed Dad, little Timmy and Janey, the nuclear family safe within its shelter. The booklets included lists of foods to be stocked—"Staples," a category made up of crackers, cookies, and pretzels; instant coffee or tea; fourteen individual-serving-size boxes of cereal, which would keep fresher than a large box (as if slightly stale Frosted Flakes would be the worst of one's worries under the circumstances); cans of beef stew, beans and franks, tuna. *"Can and bottle openers should not be forgotten!"*—the italics and exclamation point there in the original. In the back was a glossary, "Words to Know": A-Bomb, H-Bomb, Kiloton, Megaton, Ground Zero, Fireball, Blast Wind.

At the dinner table my father told us he would not build a fallout shelter. "You'd be better off dying than surviving an atomic war." I didn't say anything, but I knew. I wanted to live. I would want to live through anything.

At the beginning of the past summer, my mother had told me I was getting "too big on top" to go without a shirt. A second warning, more harsh: "Young lady, put your shirt on!"

My friends, twin classmates from third grade, spent the night at my house and wanted to see the hair growing in the region of my body we have no other words for but "you know" and "down there," and so the three of us went in the bathroom, and I lowered my blue pajama bottoms to show them.

Then the strange, rust-colored stains I found in my underpants, the summer before I turned nine. My mother took a box of sanitary napkins and a vaguely worded booklet down from the shelf in the closet of my oldest sister, who, like my next oldest sister, had not yet started menstruating. The booklet explained that my body was getting ready to have a baby. A *baby*? I was eight years old. Decades later I learned that disabled girls have a high rate of precocious puberty—for reasons no one seems to understand—and I was relieved, my early maturity no longer seemed to be one more snare laid by my stubbornly freakish body.

Between June and September of that summer, I grew four inches. My mother let down the hems of my skirts and dresses.

At night, snug abed in my room wallpapered with miniature blue flowers and blue-and-white curtains at the window, I imagined myself as a beautiful princess in leg irons held captive in a dingy cellar, with handsome warders who descended down stone steps at night to carry out cruel but nonetheless delicious tortures to my body. The next morning the sun would come up, and I would get dressed and go out into the world and be chipper and cheerful and smart and smile at everyone. In turn I would be told what a good sport I was and that President Roosevelt had had polio. Handsome men would scoop me up in their arms and call me "Princess," and carry me hither and yon.

Of course in the fairy tales there were also monsters, trolls living under the bridge, dwarves, dark men in the shadows who limp. This is the part where it gets confusing: I'm the one they call "Princess," but I limp.

At school the girls were herded into the anteroom to the nurse's office, told to remove all our clothes but our underpants for our annual physical exam. Fifteen other girls pulled off their dresses or shirts and skirts to reveal underpants and T-shirts. I unbuttoned my blouse, and there beneath it was the slightly gray hand-me-down bra from Sears I had inherited from my mother. "Anne's wearing a bra," I overheard someone whisper. Elbows were nudged into sides, furtive glances cast.

Had it really been just a year or two before that Debby's and my favorite TV show had been *The Lone Ranger*? That on Saturday mornings, playing at her house, we would check the clock often to be sure we didn't miss the show's opening—with the theme the "William Tell Overture," and the Lone Ranger's call, "Hi-yo, Silver! Away!"?

After watching *The Lone Ranger* we would play out our own scenarios. The top in our relationship, Debby always played the role of the Lone Ranger while I was stuck with being Tonto—except when she got the plum role, that of the Lone Ranger's horse, Silver, in which case I was allowed to be the Lone Ranger, straddling her back. At some point in these games we would climb atop the footrails of the two beds in her room and, pretending that they were Silver and Scout, would rub our crotches back and forth against them as we galloped across the landscape of distant mesas and chaparral, sometimes with Butch Cavendish in hot pursuit. Sometimes Cavendish would take one or the other of us prisoner and tie us up. "Butch Cavendish is taking out my wee-wee bones!" I'd holler. "Help me! Help me!" and Debby would show up with her trusty six-shooter and make short work of Butch. What did we use as a gun? I don't remember, although it must have been a substitute for a toy gun, as neither set of parents approved of toy guns and refused to buy us one, despite our badgering and the appearance of "guns," perennially at the top of our Christmas and birthday wish lists.

While a few years before it had been easy to pretend to be Tonto or the Lone Ranger, I could no longer make that imaginative leap across the divide of gender. A friend of mine who teaches kindergarten loves the ability of her students to identify, in the stories she reads to them, not just across the boundaries of gender and race but even across the species barrier. When she finishes reading them a story and asks "Who in this story is like you?" some children will cry out with delight, "The dog! I'm the dog!"

With my sisters I went to see a cartoon of the Hans Christian Andersen fairy tale *The Snow Queen*. The Snow Queen was an evil presence, made of ice, vengeful but beautiful, her angular body topped with a face that featured enormous eyes and a widow's peak. She'd kidnapped a rosy-cheeked, blond-haired child and held him prisoner in her palace made of glittering ice. I was frightened by her but drawn to her at the same time. We had a book of Hans Christian Andersen fairy tales—an old-fashioned one that might have belonged to my mother when she was a girl, or that we might have bought for a nickel or a dime at the yearly jumble sale, a book illustrated with lithographs with deeply saturated colors—indigo, rose, terra cotta—with a tissue of thin paper protecting each illustration. I was convinced that I had once seen a picture of the Snow Queen in our book, although when I looked and looked for it I couldn't find it. But still I looked and looked, certain that someday her picture would magically reappear.

We got a television. Secondhand, of course, a tiny black-and-white screen, housed in an enormous console of veneered wood, the brand name, "Majestic," written in florid script beneath the screen, an eagle with its wings spread hovering over the *J* where the dot should be. Now our house, too, had an antenna sprouting from the roof, put up by my father, to the accompaniment of a great deal of swearing. Whenever I pitch a tent or set up a Christmas tree, I remember my father's voice saying, "Goddamn it to hell . . . Jesus H. Christ," as he did those things.

I watched shows like *Route 66 and Adventures in Paradise*. In *Route 66* two clean-cut misfits drove along U.S. 66 in a red Corvette, having meaningful encounters on the way. Fair-haired Tod, played by Martin Milner, had grown up a rich kid, but after his father's sudden death, he discovered that the family wealth had disappeared: He had been left only enough money (conveniently) to buy a Corvette. His companion, dark-haired Buzz—George Maharis—was from Hell's Kitchen. You have to be of a certain age to understand the transgressive thrill of hearing the word "hell" uttered on television. Apparently Jack Kerouac had considered suing the show's producers, claiming they had ripped off *On the Road*.

Every night when I lay down in bed, I spun out elaborate fantasies in which Buzz and Tod would take a detour and drive through Hamilton, where Tod would fall in love with me—I would have morphed into a sixteen-year-old—and I would ride off with them in the Corvette, seated in the space between the two bucket seats, straddling the hand brake, I suppose. Later, as a scaffolding for my romances, I used the show *Adventures in Paradise,* another "on the road" series, although in this case the vehicle was a schooner, the *Tiki*, skippered by a brawny American named Adam Troy, and the road was the South Pacific. Adam. Buzz. Troy. Tod.

The upside to precocious puberty was that I was tall—over five feet at the age of nine. I loved being tall. When the class picture got taken, I was told to stand at the very center in the back row. When Poppy, the new girl in class, took me home after school, the first thing her mother said to me wasn't "What happened to you?" but "Goodness, you're tall!"

In March 1961, when I was nine years old, my mother and I had gone for our usual appointment at the clinic in Utica. Dr. Friedman took one look at me, shooting skyward, and said, in his taciturn way, "She needs to have surgery." He turned to one of his minions and said, "Schedule it as soon as possible." Usually I had surgery in the summer, so I wouldn't miss school. I was to have three metal staples inserted into either side of my knee to stop my left leg, that hardy sister, from outgrowing her frail twin.

Just a few weeks later I was being checked into the hospital. My mother signed a consent form for the surgery, but it was pro forma. No one thought to question doctors in those days. The only thing that gave my mother pause was the clerk's "Religion?" She hesitated for a minute— that we didn't go to church seemed shameful, bordering on anti-American—and then said, "Uh—Protestant."

No one seemed to consider the long-term effects of causing my femur and tibia to jam together at the knee. Polio was seen as a disease of children, and the effects such surgery would have on us as adults was ignored. As a result of that surgery, my legs are roughly the same length overall, although my left knee bends at such an angle that functionally, it is several inches shorter. Years later, as I sat on an exam table in a pale blue paper gown, an orthopedist took one look at my left leg, let out a low, gee-whiz whistle, and said, "Well, I don't need an X-ray to see what's gone wrong there." A few minutes later, when I mentioned pain, he said, "Yeah, well, that oughta hurt."

After I'd been checked in to the hospital, my mother left. I was all right at first, but soon it was nap time, marked by the roller shades being pulled down, which made the light dim but without giving the comforting oblivion of night: an artificial, extended twilight. I could not be ordered to bed, as I was already in bed, but I was told to be quiet, to rest. Sleep was impossible. I became acutely aware of the institutional ugliness of the room: the metal hospital bed, painted white, the paint chipped and grimy, with railings on either side, like a crib; the nightstand next to it, in a modern material that was supposed to look like wood but did not, into which my mother had packed the few forlorn things I had brought with me; the walls, painted in dim institutional shades of green or beige. Nothing was right, not the sounds of the city, so different from the background noise of the country, with the distant croaks of toads, the rumble of a tractor from a nearby field, the rustling of the wind moving through weeds and trees, the lowing of cattle, the steady hum from dishwasher or washing machine or clothes dryer—one of those machines was always running in our house—the voices of my sisters and brother. Those sounds I was never aware of, except now, in their absence.

The sheets I lay on were harsh. My mother was so thrifty that our sheets were soft and worn. If the fabric ripped, weakened after so many usings and washings, she stitched them up. In the winter she dried them in the dryer, but in the summer she hung them on the line outside, fastening them with wooden clothespins. Even in the winter they held on to some of the battered softness of sun and wind from having been dried outdoors. The cotton aged into a thin, almost silklike texture. Favorite T-shirts I've had for years and years get this same almost-gossamer quality just before they go through the equivalent of a final illness, emerging from the dryer one last time with holes where the fabric has finally given way.

The sheets at the hospital were different, thick and stiff. Unlike the rumpled sheets on my bed at home, these had not only been pressed in a mangle but then had been made up with official hospital corners so that they were sharp and unyielding. When my aunt Dorothy, who trained as a nurse, came to visit, she not only cleaned our oven—my mother hated to clean the oven—but gave us lessons in how to make our beds with the geometric precision she learned in nursing school. Making our beds with hospital corners seemed fun for a day or two, but then we drifted back to my mother's way of doing things and thought of housework not as an art but as a necessary evil.

Did I miss my mother? I missed everything. I knew the hospital routines. After nap time, a rickety-wheeled cart would come clattering along the linoleum floor. We would be offered our choice of graham crackers or saltines, milk or orange juice. I knew that if I had the orange juice it would be straight from a can, and taste nothing like the remixed frozen orange juice at home. Since I was used to the mix of milk and Starlac my mother gave us at home, the milk here would be cloying and too thick. I wouldn't have the sensation of real glass pressed against my lips, but that of the unbreakable Melamac cups used at the hospital.

I was aware of tears starting to gather in my eyes. How could I be homesick when I was so old?

The last time I was in the hospital, when I was six years old, my father appeared once during visiting hours instead of my mother. He was there to tell me I was upsetting my mother by crying when she came to visit, and that I must stop.

"I can't help it," I said.

"You're not crying now," he pointed out. I couldn't tell him that I didn't feel like crying when I saw him. I felt like crying only when I saw my mother. I didn't miss him the way I missed her.

"You are making her too sad," he said.

My father wasn't the only one to reprimand me. When I was six, one of the nurses told me that if I didn't stop crying for my mother, I was going to be sent to another hospital where children were never allowed to see their mothers. Of course I only wailed louder at the thought of that. Some nurses pointed out that other children—some of whose parents hardly ever came to visit them—didn't cry. Now I think of those children, resigned to their profound losses, and realize that they were so depressed they had ceased to cry.

I wasn't alone in being discouraged from showing normal childhood emotions. Nancy Frick recalled that for years before she had polio, she was subject to nightmares. When she woke up crying, her mother would comfort her:

> When I entered the hospital the nightmares continued. There was a night nurse at the hospital who did not like my crying and did not comfort me because I sometimes would awaken the other patients. When she came to my bed she would say in a very threatening voice, "You stop crying or you are going to be sorry." She frightened me for two reasons: I knew I couldn't control the nightmares and I didn't know what she would do to me when I cried again. Then, one night I found out. I awoke crying from a nightmare; she came in and said, "I told you not to do this or you were going to be sorry." She pulled me in my hospital bed into a walk in [*sic*] linen closet, turned off the light, closed the door, locked it and left me there until morning.

Marilyn Rogers, hospitalized at the Sister Kenny Institute in 1949, was almost killed as punishment for crying. In pain because the collar of her iron lung was rubbing against her skin, she was told by a "frustrated and overworked" nurse to "stop crying. She said she would turn my respirator off if I didn't stop crying. When she did I passed out immediately." Rogers's life was saved because some assistants turned the iron lung back on.

I am drawn to the writings of the great Italian intellectual, Antonio Gramsci, who spent most of his adult life imprisoned under Mussolini's Fascist regime, for many reasons; but I feel a particular resonance between his prison experiences and mine in hospitals. Several years after his arrest he wrote about the mental state he had been forced to develop in prison, which I think must have been like that of those children who did not cry, who were held up to me as exemplars:

> They say that the sea beyond thirty meters of depth is always immobile. I have sunk to a depth of at least twenty meters. I am immersed in the layer that moves only when storms of a certain size, well above normal, are unleashed. But I feel that I am sinking deeper and deeper and I can lucidly see the moment in which, by imperceptible degrees, I will reach the level of absolute immobility, where even the most formidable storms no longer make themselves felt.

What Gramsci was describing was the process of institutionalization, the psyche dulling itself in response to the demands of the institution. But institutionalization doesn't affect only the inmates; it also affects the personalities of those who work in such institutions. They, too, can become numb, submissive to routines, emotionally blunted.

In the days before press-on pads, an elastic belt with metal prongs on either end was used to anchor sanitary napkins. The nurse hoisting the belt over my legs, my left one encased in a plaster cast, seemed faintly disgruntled and perhaps also disgusted that I was menstruating at nine. "My daughter's sixteen, and she doesn't have her period yet." She said it as if there were a supply of menarches waiting in a storehouse somewhere and, stretching in front of it, a long line of expectant, nearly adolescent girls waiting their turn to be doled out the gift of menarche, and I'd pushed my way to the front, snatched up the one that was meant for her daughter, and made off with it clutched tightly to my chest. I wanted to tell her that I would be more than happy to take the elasticized belt, the booklet from the Kotex corporation, the bloody pads themselves, wrap them up in brightly colored wrapping paper, festoon the gift with ribbons, add an enormous gold bow, and present the entire lot to her poor deprived daughter. She could have it, and I could go back to running around bare chested and catching crayfish in the creek and building forts.

When I came home from the hospital, I didn't sleep in my upstairs bedroom, where I used to wake up early and look out over the six maple trees in the front yard, and then across Glen Denmark's fields to the line of willow trees next to the creek that ran alongside the Crouches' house, fresh shoots sprouting from their chopped-off trunks. Instead I slept in the downstairs room that had become the television room.

My mother had started working, teaching English to the sons and daughters of farmers in nearby Earleville. She taught the morning classes and her friend Posey Smith the afternoon ones, so I was alone every morning, stretched out on the maroon daybed. I got up only to go to the bathroom.

Did I eat breakfast in the kitchen with my sisters and brother before they went off to school, at the wooden table we had dented by banging our knives and forks against it, chanting "We want to eat! We want to eat!" as if we were convicts in a Jimmy Cagney movie about to start a riot in the prison mess hall? (Oh, my poor mother!) Did I walk into the kitchen, leaning on my wooden crutches? Or did my mother bring me a bowl of cereal, a paper napkin, a glass of orange juice on a plastic tray? I try to conjure up the scene, but the tray I see is an orange plastic rectangle, the sort from school cafeterias—and I know we wouldn't have had one like that. The early morning hours are blank space. I can fill them in only through supposition.

I know I must have heard, through the walls, my mother padding down the stairs in her slippers in the morning, the sounds of water running in the kitchen, the refrigerator door opening and closing as she made our breakfasts and lunches, heard her calling up the stairs, first a general, "Kids! Time to get up!" A few minutes later she would call out the name of whoever had failed to appear: "Sandra! Are you up? Answer me so I know you're up!" And then she called my father, "Jack! Your breakfast is almost ready!" Would she have let me sleep in, since there was no reason for me to get up? Or did she wake me up, trying to preserve the normality of a routine, not wanting me to awaken alone in an empty house?

Maybe she just opened the door, allowing the noises of the house to drift in. Maybe I heard her setting the brown paper lunch sacks—four instead of the usual five—with names written on them with Magic Marker on the table, the clink of pennies set in front of each—milk money. Three cents for my brother and younger sister, because milk was cheaper in first and second grades; four cents—or was it a nickel?—for the older kids. The morning's tempo must have increased as eight o'clock—the hour when the school bus arrived—came closer. "Susan, the bus is going to be here in fifteen minutes." "Where's my white blouse?" "Did you look in your closet?" "You can't got to school without breakfast." "The school bus will be here in three minutes!" The noises must have reached a crescendo, and then there would have been silence as the last person to leave shut the door.

Was I lonely? Or was there the excitement of being home alone? In those halcyon days before we knew about AIDS and herpes and Ebola and SARS, people used to talk about "finding the cure for the common cold," the last frontier in the battle against contagious illness. I loved the excitement of being in the house alone when I had a cold and hoped the cure never got found. I would get to stay home and gorge myself on the usually forbidden TV until I felt that peculiar sensation in my head that was not quite a headache—there's a German expression for that feeling, "square eyes." With this so much longer stretch of time had the thrill long since worn off?

And who was the last person to leave?

My father, of course. There are things I haven't so much forgotten as not thought about in years or decades. The paper sacks with our names written on them in Magic Marker in which we used to carry our lunches to school. The pennies stacked in front of each of our bags. The fights my father and oldest sister used to have every morning after my mother had returned to work and so left the house early, and my father was the one to see us off to school in the morning.

Every morning, they had the same fight:

"I won't have my daughter going out in public looking like a goddamn tramp."

"Daddy," Sandra pleaded. "No one wears their skirts down below their knees anymore."

"Is this how you were brought up?" he yelled. "To go along with the crowd? Just do what other people are doing?"

The words "tramp" and "whore," the threat of violence always in the air. I knew that my sister looked like every other seventh-grade girl on the school bus, with her navy blue knee socks and pleated kilt and white blouse with the Peter Pan collar and the fake gold circle pin.

My brother asked my father, "How come we never have any money?"

"Because your goddamn sister Sandra spends all our money on Elvis Presley records."

Sandra had to pay fines when she left her clothes on the bathroom floor. Fifteen cents for every piece of clothing on the bathroom floor, and my father had found four things.

"Your goddamn skirt, your blouse, your panties, and your brassiere."

We were at the dinner table, staring at our plates, gingerly picking up peas with our forks, trying to eat, trying not to cry.

"But Daddy—" Sandra said.

"Don't you 'But Daddy' me. Your skirt, your blouse, your bra, your panties. Four times fifteen, that's sixty cents. Sixty."

"Daddy, I don't have any money."

"That's not my problem. That's not my goddamn problem."

"You haven't given me my allowance in three weeks. Give me my allowance, and then—"

Tears welled in Sandra's eyes and my mother looked at her and muttered, "Don't cry. Don't make things worse."

"Your skirt, your blouse, your bra, your panties. Four times fifteen, that's sixty cents."

"Daddy, I'll pay the fine when you give me my allowance."

"I am so goddamn sick of hearing you whine and whine. You owe your fine, and you have to pay it."

"Give me my allowance."

"Do you think you can go before a judge, the judge orders a fine, and you can blame someone else who hasn't paid you? No, you'll get sent to goddamn jail."

"Well, but, Jack," my mother said, in her most soothing voice, "I think Sandra has a point."

My father glared at my mother, pounded on the table with both of his fists: "Whose side are you on?"

I knew that these fights were not about the length of my sister's skirts or about Elvis Presley records or clothes left on the bathroom floor. I knew they were about something else, about that mysterious part of my body called "down there" and "you know." And I know that it is my braces and crutches that protect me from his sexualized rage.

My sense of my sexual self grows inside of me like a seedling unexposed to light: translucent, fragile, peculiar.

When I am in my forties, I go to a dinner party. One of the guests tells the story of his fourteen-year-old daughter who had just gotten her first bikini. She had put it on, and gone out in the yard to shoot baskets. "Look, Dad! Look!" she had called, dribbling the ball, leaping toward the basket. "Dad, look!" And he mimed the way he had looked at her, his eyes partly covered by his hand. He repeated the tentative way he had said, "Yeah, that's great, honey, great," while he and his wife both laughed.

I tell this story over and over again in therapy.

That is how you could feel about a daughter's emerging sexuality: proud and embarrassed. You could be drawn to her, and wary of your attraction to her, but in a way you could laugh about at a dinner party.

Among the classes my father taught at Colgate was "Child and Adolescent Development." The description in the course catalog read, "Principles of the child's mental, physical, emotional and social development; the influence and responsibilities of the home, the school, the community and other social agencies in meeting the basic human needs of the child and the adolescent."

Everything my father knew, all his knowledge, all the books he had read: None of those did anything to help him, to rescue him from the wild near-madness that had him in its grip.

As I lay there, alone, in the empty house, sometimes my boredom became almost palpable, a dense gray substance surrounding me, stretching beyond the horizon, so viscous that when I tried to free myself from it, tendrils of it clung to my body.

Sometimes, instead of being a close cousin to depression, boredom took on another cast. Lying there, doing nothing, waiting, was the polar opposite of the Yankee diligence that formed the foundation of my family's life. When this shift happened, instead of looking out over an ocean of infinite, solid gray, I gazed out on an open field of unending imaginative possibilities.

Since televisions in Hamilton could pick up only a single channel and the morning news and quiz shows bored me, I must have read during those first few hours.

I know that sometimes I flipped through a history of English costume from the fourteenth to the nineteenth century, with full-color lithographs. I didn't much like to look at the pictures from the 1300s and 1400s. The foolscap of the jesters, the snoods covering the women's hair, the ermine capes in which the nobility was attired, all made the figures seem so distant that it was hard for me to imagine that these people had once lived. Their lives had been as important to them as mine was to me, and now they were not just dead but so remote that their lives lay beyond my imaginative powers. No matter how hard I tried to keep the thought from entering my mind, it seemed to come in unbidden—someday the clothes I wore would seem as strange and ridiculous as the horned headdresses and belled and pointed shoes of that day did to me. A description of clothing from Chaucer's *Canterbury Tales* was quoted, among them this description of the Monk's costume: "He hadde of gold ywrought a curious pyn; A love-knotte in the gretter ende ther was."

When I referred to this as Old English, my mother had laughed and said, no, this was Middle English. She dug out her college copy of *Beowulf* and showed it to me, the letters glyphs and the language impenetrable—*that* was Old English. It was not just the clothes I wore that would someday become ancient, but the very language I spoke, the language I used to ward off my despair and powerlessness.

Further along in the book, the figures came more closely to resemble the illustrations in fairy tales or Disney cartoons, and I was less troubled by them. Fashions for enormous ostrich feather plumes came and went, as did the elaborate lace cuffs and cravats of the Restoration.

I read and reread titillating passages of this book. In the late sixteenth century those surrounding the royal court had engaged in "ultrasophisticated and immoral behaviour." Although I understood the concepts both of "sophisticated" and "immoral," I had only the vaguest notion of how this might actually translate into behavior among the fashionable. The vocabulary of Queen Elizabeth I "would probably shock even the broadest-minded of men of to-day." What had she said? Words worse than "hell" and "damn"? Something more than the "Kiss my ass" Mr. Crouch said? But what could those words be?

And I read: "King James abandoned himself to drink and vice, and the court became a scene of carousing and debauchery." Because the little I knew about the act of sexual intercourse had been presented to me in terms of making a baby, it seemed not naughty and pleasurable but an activity that my parents carried out in the same spirit with which they put up the storm windows or cleaned out the gutters. I couldn't imagine that the aforesaid "vice . . . and debauchery" were connected with the little I knew of intercourse. "Vice . . . and debauchery" remained mysterious, although tinged with an enticing wickedness. The mystery bled into other words in the book whose meanings I did not know: "cravat . . . turban . . . French cuffs . . . pelisse." I would not have wanted to look them up in the dictionary. If I had learned that a *pelisse* was a kind of cloak and that "cravat" was a synonym for "necktie," those words would have deflated, ending up as empty and dull as the words "storm window" or "gutter."

And then, finally, at eleven o'clock, *The Million Dollar Movie* came on.

When I went back to visit Hamilton, I checked into the Colgate Inn. It had been a long drive up from New York City: I plopped myself down on the bed, and then, a few minutes later, wiggled down to the foot of the bed, leaned forward to open the armoire with the TV inside, picked up the remote, the card that listed the channels. There were nearly a hundred of them: MTV and Animal Planet, sports channels, CNN.

Even when the television was working perfectly, the black and white pixels forming the picture were clearly visible. Often something would go kerflooey. The picture might start to roll, and Garbo's famous face would become elongated, looking like my mother's did when I saw it through the postsurgical hallucinogenic fog of ether. Or ghostly images from other channels might move across the screen. I'd have to make my way to the television set, leaning heavily on my crutches, and fiddle with the knobs marked "horizontal" and "vertical." If that didn't work, I'd whack the side of the TV, which might make the picture snap into shape—or might make things worse.

I watched Joan Crawford and Greta Garbo, Rita Hayworth and Jeanette MacDonald. I could not imagine myself as a woman like the mothers around me in Hamilton, so perhaps I would become like the women in these movies. I'd wear glamorous outfits, and men would strew flowers at my feet.

In *Mata Hari,* the story of a female spy during World War I who bewitched men and led them to betray their native land, one of the other female spies turned out to be a double agent and so had to be done away with. The chief German spy called out "Jacques!" and disability limped onto the screen. The word "limp" is called upon to cover so many differing gaits, from a stiff-legged hesitation to his clumping lurch. All the viewer saw of Jacques as he entered the frame was a close-up of his lower legs. One of his legs was shortened; his shoe had an enormous wedge on the bottom of it. Off he gallumphed after Carlotta, the spy who had betrayed the spymasters; Carlotta screamed—she was not only going to die, she was going to die the sort of terrible death that would be inflicted by someone twisted in body and spirit.

And in *Grand Hotel,* one of the very first shots was of a facially disfigured doctor, who speaks the first lines of dialogue, weary and Zen-like: "Grand Hotel. Always the same. People come, people go. Nothing ever happens."

In *Grand Hotel,* Garbo played the role of a jaded ballerina, Grusinskaya. As I look at that name written on the page, it conjures up a dumpy careworn woman, perhaps leaning on a mop, who would snort her name with a guttural frankness: "Grusinskaya." No, you have to imagine the way Garbo said it, flinging back her head and trilling the *r,* caressing the penultimate syllable, allowing her intonation to rise and fall and then rise again; finally giving a histrionic shrug of her lanky shoulders.

I didn't know that the characters who populated the Grand Hotel were all types: I had never before seen the roué—Baron von Geigern, played by John Barrymore—long on charm and short on cash; this was the first time I'd encountered the wily stenographer—Flämmchen (Little Flame), Joan Crawford in the days before her face was frozen into a mask of pseudo-youthfulness—of loose morals and a good heart. Nor had I seen before the character played by Wallace Beery—was ever an actor more aptly named?—the bulky, self-satisfied German industrialist. As for the prima donna behaving—well, like a prima donna—Garbo's character seemed to be my sister soul, when she spoke of her terrible unhappiness, the temptations of suicide. In her satin peignoir, reclining on satin sheets, she declared, "I can't dance tonight," pronouncing the word "dance" as if it were polysyllabic. "Pearls are cold, everything's cold. . . . It's not stage fright—it's something more." A soul in torment—and those heartless impresarios, speaking of contracts and obligations—they were even worse than my mother when she told me to quit moping around.

I had to do a head transplant onto the character played by John Barrymore so that he could have a role in my fantasies. With his brilliantined hair, pencil mustache, and carefully groomed eyebrows, he seemed positively repulsive, the kind of man who might leer at you from the cover of a magazine called *Swank* or *Rascal*. I imagined instead the face of the blond and gentle Tab Hunter. Tab Hunter would fall in love with me as the baron had fallen in love with the prima ballerina; we would kiss, as they kissed in the movies, our mouths tightly shut; our lovemaking would be vague and spiritual and fluidless.

If there had been a real Grand Hotel in Berlin, it would have been bombed to rubble and dust, perhaps a few shards of its walls would have risen like tragic stalagmites out of the rock-strewn landscape of postwar Berlin. But it had never existed; it had been born only in the imagination of novelist Vicki Baum and then made flesh in the MGM studios. And then all trickery and deceit: antique gold paint slathered on plaster, the magnificent spiral staircase, shot from above, nothing but a cardboard-and-balsa miniature.

THE MAKINGS OF A DISEASE

I

The Uses of Illness

What interests does a disease serve? The question at first seems an odd one, and our first response might be: Disease serves no one's interest. Illness is a universal evil, something to be fought against, eradicated. Although it is true that being an enemy is a function of a sort—and surely every society has needed to have an antagonist of one kind or another. The gentlest brotherhood of Buddhist monks living in Bhutan or Nepal does battle with the temptations of the world of illusion, a pacific sort of battle but a battle nonetheless.

In her brilliant essays *Illness As Metaphor* and *AIDS* and *Its Metaphors,* Susan Sontag discussed how societies have made metaphoric use of diseases. In particular she showed how certain illnesses—tuberculosis, cancer, and AIDS—have not only had a whole series of meanings attached to them but have been used as overarching social metaphors. Tuberculosis was the emblematic disease of the romantic period, with its images of youth expiring in a fevered poetic bloom, like candles with untrimmed wicks burning wildly before dying out too soon. Later, cancer came to be seen as an inexorably spreading blot, formed from our sins—whether those were personal failings or the evils of unchecked industrialism. Cancer became a shorthand for describing whatever threatened us: Drugs were a cancer, spreading insidiously across the land, or the American empire was a cancer.

Sontag noted that AIDS had come to be seen as the punishment for licentiousness, the ultimate proof that we have "gone too far." I think that now, nearly two decades after Sontag wrote *AIDS and Its Metaphors,* the meaning of AIDS is shifting. It is increasingly seen as a disease of the third world, particularly of Africa, and is read as a sign of the (supposedly) intractable divisions between rich countries and the global south, the impoverished nations of Africa, Asia, and Latin America. Sontag wrote that not only did AIDS come to have meanings, but that in the era of AIDS, metaphors relating to viruses abound. Speaking of destructive computer programs that are hidden within a seemingly innocuous program—better known, of course, as computer "viruses"—she wrote: "It is perhaps not surprising that the newest transforming element in the modern world, computers, should be borrowing metaphors drawn from our newest transforming illness."

Sontag stated that her aim in these two essays was "not to confer meaning, which is the traditional purpose of literary endeavor, but to deprive something of meaning." But making meaning is fundamental to being human. We may look up at the night sky and see Orion and Andromeda. Or we may see the effects of light pollution. Or we may see our human insignificance. We read the night sky, just as we read disability itself, along with individual diseases. No disease can be stripped of its metaphoric meanings until we are left with some pure, naked disease, the illness's true self. I want to understand the multiple meanings that make up the disease—how those readings were changed over time, the impacts that the meanings had and continue to have, the social forces that shaped them.

II

Made for Each Other

To consider the making of polio, let's return to that early mass epidemic in New York in 1916. In June, before the epidemic broke, the fearsome heat of summer had not yet set in. It wasn't just discomfort and lassitude that threatened city dwellers on torrid summer days. "[Summer] is the harvest season for death's reaper," wrote reformer Charles Stelzle, looking back on the early days of the twentieth century. Cholera and yellow fever seemed to thrive in the dank air, the miasma of city odors. In the year 1916 the infant mortality rate was eighty-eight per thousand live births. Of course, the death rate wasn't evenly spread across classes. Tenement dwellers were more at risk than those who lived in Park Avenue mansions, but no one was safe in the days before penicillin, when every ear or lung infection might turn into something deadly. The reality of death may have been roughly one in ten, but the threat was omnipresent. Nearly every time a child fell ill, death was a possibility.

Dr. Haven Emerson was New York's health commissioner in 1916. Emerson—yes, as in Ralph Waldo—America's eminent philosopher and poet was this Dr. Emerson's great-uncle; Haven Emerson came from a long line of Puritans, contrarians, and patricians. Long-faced, tall, gangly—later, when his hair turned white, he bore a more-than-passing resemblance to Ichabod Crane. Haven Emerson, unlike his noble ancestor, rooted his approach to the world not in sympathy, but in clarity. He had graduated from the finest universities—Harvard College, Columbia's College of Physicians and Surgeons. Having abandoned Boston for New York—Athens for Rome, some would say—he was ready to go out and grapple with ill health, do battle with disease, wrestle it to the ground.

It would be ghoulish to paint him as welcoming the epidemic, although the new disease and the new profession of public health do seem to have been made for each other, as if they were engaged in a process of mutual self-creation. Consider this singular fact: Before the twentieth century nearly one-half of all children died before they reached adolescence. In the nineteenth century, medical science was of such poor quality that Oliver Wendell Holmes, himself a physician, said: "If the whole *materia medica,* as now used, could be sunk to the bottom of the sea, it would be all the better for mankind—and all the worse for the fishes."

By the middle of the nineteenth century, pediatrics was emerging as a distinct specialty, although most families undoubtedly had little access to physicians of any sort and continued to confront childhood illness with a combination of prayer, tenderness, traditional remedies—and resignation. As the nineteenth century turned into the twentieth, the profession of pediatrics began to come into its own, with the establishment of medical journals specifically devoted to child health and disease. The four-volume *Cyclopedia of Diseases of Children,* published in 1890, was followed two decades later by an even more massive "system of pediatrics," which ran to ten thousand pages. Significantly, the profession of pediatrics became concerned not only with treatment of disease but with broader issues of overall child well-being, including hygiene, nutrition, growth, and development. Indeed, the new practice of pediatrics extended its reach far beyond what is ordinarily thought of as the medical sphere, positing itself as the source of authority on everything from diapering to the physical layout of the nursery. This medicalization of infancy and childhood is now so deeply ingrained that the fact that what many still regard as the bible of American child rearing was written by a pediatrician, Dr. Benjamin Spock, seems completely unremarkable.

As medical surveillance of the child increased, the profession of pediatrics extended its reach beyond care of children as individuals to broader social arenas: "They advised judges and penal institutions on delinquency, they informed educators on children's health and its maintenance, they lobbied politicians for greater funding for child welfare." This marked a significant shift in power to men—since the vast majority of pediatricians were male—and a professionalization of knowledge that had previously been diffused and shared.

Polio was an ideal disease for the newly emerging professions of pediatrics and public health to focus on. Tuberculosis was more common, but the ubiquity of tuberculosis made it harder to formulate public health campaigns concerning the disease. Resignation, rather than panic, was often the response to a case of TB. We exist in a state of truce with disease; we have certain expectations of it. (When I was in my late thirties I was aware of how wrong it seemed that, because of AIDS, I had lost more friends than my elderly parents: It was not the way my compact with illness was supposed to play out.)

As part of the new practices of public health, the doctor would not wait for patients to summon him. He would go out and intervene actively in the community. With fear of this strange new disease as the goal, Dr. Emerson and the health department could roll up their sleeves and get to work.

Dr. Emerson began to enlist an army for health, gathered not for the taking of lives as in war, but for saving them from disease. DEFENSE LEAGUE OF 21,000 CITIZENS FIGHTS PARALYSIS read the headline in the July 9, 1916, *New York Times*. The streets of the city were patrolled by members of this Home Defense League, organized to assist the police in any time of crisis. Accompanied by policemen, they searched streets and homes for violations of the sanitary code, although the article also noted that their actions might well be ineffective: "In epidemics of typhoid fever and most other disease, the health authorities know exactly what to do. But fighting infantile paralysis consists largely in doing everything that seems effective in the hope that some of the measures will be effective." To extend the military metaphor, the germ that caused infantile paralysis was a guerrilla, elusive, invisible, striking in seemingly random fashion, hiding amid a population unaware of its presence.

These "volunteer vigilante forces," as the *Times* described them, included "prominent men and men of affairs," some of whom reported to work in elegant summer garb. They made their way through city streets searching for sanitary-code violators, who were brought into court and fined. The health department and others mobilized in the war against infantile paralysis must have seemed to be an army occupying immigrant neighborhoods.

Along with public health officials, these volunteers undertook intensive "house-to-house inspections" in immigrant neighborhoods, seeking to uncover cases of the disease, enforce quarantine, and instruct individuals on proper sanitation of apartments and rooms, food preparation, and personal hygiene. At the same time reports were made to the proper city departments about "bad housing conditions, unclean tenements, overcrowding, violations of the food laws, dirty streets, cellars and yards, garbage and litter, disorderly or illegally occupied premises, and other nuisances."

With more than a bit of bureaucratic hedging, the health department's *Monograph on the Epidemic of Poliomyelitis,* published in 1917, noted that the department's nurses "were fairly well received in a large percentage of instances." One can infer the unstated—that in many instances the attentions of the nurses were *not* well received. Residents of the Fort Greene section of Brooklyn protested against physicians and inspectors being sent into their neighborhood, fearing—not without reason—that they might be carrying "the germ" from house to house as they went about their rounds. The *Monograph* also noted that "results obtained among adults were largely due to fear of authority and the force of the department and not to voluntary action on their part."

In fact, sometimes physical force on the part of the police was necessary to remove children to the hospital, and there were threats of court action against those who attempted to hide cases from health authorities. The Department of Health reminded the *Monograph*'s readers: "It is perhaps unnecessary to recall the fact that the powers vested in the Board of

Health to adopt the provisions of the Sanitary Code have been repeatedly sustained by the highest courts of this State."

On the same day that the *Times* ran its article about the defense league taking to the streets, a story in the *New York Tribune,* which catered to a less elite readership, was headlined: "Mothers of Plague Sufferers Battle to Keep Their Babies." The story painted a vivid portrait of women screaming for help (most often in a language other than English) as their children were snatched from their arms. An ambulance driver reported that brute force was necessary to remove children from their parents in nearly all immigrant neighborhoods. The driver was quoted on events from the previous day:

> We brought in eight babies this morning on one trip, and in every case we had to get policemen before we were able to put the baby in the ambulance. Without a policeman we went down to . . . a district inhabited chiefly by immigrant Poles. The doctor argued for twenty minutes with one father before the man finally told his wife to give us the baby. And when the child was taken to the ambulance the mother screamed and fought. Then the father, shrieking that we were trying to steal his child, snatched the baby and ran into the house.
>
> I drove the ambulance away when a threatening crowd began to gather, and in Twentieth Street we picked up two policemen, who went with us throughout the rest of the trip. Everywhere we went we had trouble, and only the presence of the policemen kept us from being mobbed. In the Italian district . . . we were denounced as "Black Hands," come to steal babies and hold them for ransom or murder them.

The ambulance driver's day was not over yet, however. At the home of one suspected case, one of the two policeman managed to come up behind the mother and snatch her infant from her while the second officer held the father downstairs. The mother "pursued him, sobbing and shrieking, and neighbors began pouring into the street from every tenement, some of them carrying bricks and clubs."

The health department allowed infantile paralysis patients to be treated at home, provided that a number of conditions were met, including the hiring of a "special attendant, who must observe quarantine regulations, do no cooking, and avoid contact with household children," and a "special room for patient and attendant." These measures were completely impossible for the poor. Although treatments were given to hospitalized patients, they were essentially useless and may have been harmful. The only real benefit might have been not to the hospitalized but to the broader community, from isolation of the affected. Even that benefit is dubious, given that the disease was largely spread by nonparalytic cases and carriers who never themselves developed a clinical illness.

The health authorities did not comprehend the attitude of Southern Italian immigrants toward hospitals. *Pozz' fini in dint ospedale*, "May you end your days in a hospital," was a curse. In Italy those who were forced to resort to hospitals for health care were outcasts—lepers, vagrants—who had no family to care for them. Hospitals, with their bureaucratic routines, their strange foods, and their incomprehensible language; their barring children from the warmth and comfort of their mothers, seemed the very antithesis of what was needed to restore health. On this last point contemporary thought agrees with Italian folk wisdom. Few now doubt the enormous trauma that ensues when children are separated from loving contact with their parents.

One nurse, who had been investigating supposed cases of infantile paralysis in an Italian neighborhood of Brooklyn and sending children to hospitals, received a "Black Hand" letter. One newspaper account even stated that it was written in blood. "If you report any more of our babies to the Board of Health we will kill you and nobody will know what happened to you. Keep off our streets and don't report our homes and we will do you no harm." The nurse, Mrs. Anna Henry, was thereafter escorted about by police officers. Dr. William J. Burns, the health officer of Oyster Bay, received a death threat from what the *Times* reported as "the Italian colony." The only hospital in the area was located within the Italian neighborhood, and Dr. Burns was warned that if he continued to bring infantile paralysis patients there from other parts of Long Island he would be killed and the hospital would be burned. That was only an opening volley in the battle between locals and health authorities in Oyster Bay.

Italian custom decreed that windows should be tightly shut at night to keep evil spirits from entering the home. Perhaps this belief derived from living in a region where malaria was endemic. Evil spirits—in the form of *Anopheles gambiae*, the mosquito that carries malaria—can indeed enter through open windows at night. To native-born health workers, fresh air was valued in large part because it was seen as the ultimate remedy for tuberculosis. Tuberculars were sent to mountains and deserts where the fresh air was assumed to be health giving and consumed as much of it as possible by spending long hours of both the day and the night outdoors. It was assumed that fresh air was a palliative against any number of ills.

The Italian word *malaria* tells a completely opposite story about air. Literally translated as "bad air," it suggests that miasmas and airborne pollution—not in our contemporary industrial pollution but in the biblical sense of defilement and uncleanliness, whether moral or physical—were a cause of illness. One social worker reported:

> In one house I went into the only window was not only shut, but the cracks were stuffed with rags, so that the "disease" could not come in. You can imagine what the dark, dirty room was like; the babies had no clothes on, and were so wet and hot that they looked as if they had been dipped in oil, and the flies were sticking all over them.

In the face of the polio epidemic, native-born middle-class nurses struggled to do what to them was the logical thing—throw open the windows so that the health-giving air could enter, while the Italian mothers struggled just as valiantly to do the logical thing and shut out the malignant, disease-carrying air.

III

Overcoming

In 1875 Jean-Martin Charcot, the French neurologist—most widely known now for having been a mentor of Sigmund Freud—heard a case presented to the Parisian Society of Biology. The left side of a young man had been paralyzed by polio when he was an infant. He had made a partial recovery and become a tanner. As part of his occupation he pulled heavy wet hides from vats in which they had been treated. By the age of seventeen he was experiencing fatigue and weakness in both the arm and leg of his right side. This is apparently the first published article about postpolio syndrome.

From 1875 until 1900 twenty-four articles appeared in European medical journals describing late-onset weakness and sometimes out-and-out atrophy—muscle wasting—as a result of earlier polio. In 1903 Charles Potts wrote the first article for an American medical journal on the late effects of polio; nearly two dozen additional articles were published describing these late effects prior to 1936. Articles in medical journals described not just increasing muscle weakness but related respiratory problems. But as polio became a disease that could be "overcome," this knowledge of the late effects of polio was suppressed and forgotten, as it did not fit in with the narrative about polio being a disease that could be conquered through individual will and hard work.

I go to the library at UC Berkeley to see one of these very early articles for myself. The librarian double-checks to make sure that the volume isn't so brittle that it's kept in a locked case. No, it is on the open shelves, the librarian tells me. The original binding must have been in bad shape, though, because it has been rebound in nondescript library binding. Some of the other volumes of the French journal in which Charcot published his early work are bound as they must originally have been—in thin leather covers etched with gold decorations, the endpapers marbled, although the bindings are beginning to flake away. On those old volumes a white sticker gives the call number, written in an ornate hand with a fountain pen.

When I open the century-old volume, the edges of the pages have turned sepia and grown brittle. Although my French is anything but fluent, I can do a rough translation: "X, nineteen years old, had at the age of six months convulsions and fever, followed by paralysis of the left side. By the age of seven he had partially recovered the use of his arm and leg. At the age of fourteen he became an apprentice tanner. His health was always good; he was strong, tall, vigorous. After two years he experienced weakness in his right arm and fatigue."

I also pulled a contemporary volume of the same journal off the shelf. Although the text is in both English and French, the text is equally incomprehensible in either language: "Increased expression of IL6 mRNA is found within the glomeruli in mesangioproliferative glomerulonephritis and IL6 protein is detectable in proliferating mesangial areas."

We don't think of medical knowledge as simply being forgotten, as having been stuffed in closets and then lost. But that is what happened with awareness of what has now come to be known as postpolio syndrome.

Partly it was the sheer bulk of the known, but I think it was more than information glut, the impossibility of knowing all that is to be known. Knowledge of postpolio syndrome disappeared because it no longer fitted with the story of the disease. If the narrative was one of overcoming, if we were supposed to fight our way back, if not to normalcy to as close to normalcy as possible, how could we imagine that the process would, after a certain point, reverse itself? Knowledge of postpolio syndrome disappeared until the late 1970s, when

... reports began to surface that people who had recovered from paralytic polio decades earlier were developing unexpected health problems such as excessive fatigue, pain in muscles and joints and, most alarming of all, new muscle weakness. . . . [T]he initial response by many physicians was that the problems were not real. For a time they were dealing with a cluster of symptoms that had no name—and without a name there was, in essence, no disease. Having a name—even if imprecise and misleading as to causation—at least confers an element of credibility.

And what of those hundreds of thousands of survivors of the polio virus who lived during that period of time before the syndrome was given a name? Some of them, surely, must have died in their sleep when their weakened respiratory muscles were no longer able to function as they once had. Others must have been told that it was all in their heads, sent to psychiatrists, prescribed antidepressants and tranquilizers. Still others found themselves mistakenly diagnosed with other neurological ailments, such as amyotrophic lateral sclerosis, or Lou Gehrig's disease. Perhaps, in some sense, they were the lucky ones, because they must have been relieved when, having been given a diagnosis that amounted to a death sentence, they found themselves outliving their predicted quick demise. Others must have kept up their *I-think-I-can, I-think-I-can, I-think-I-can* behavior, going until they dropped in their tracks.

PROVIDENCE

When I was ten my father was hired by Brown University, and we moved from Hamilton to Providence, Rhode Island. We lived on Larch Street, which runs perpendicular to Hope Street. Hope begins at swanky Blackstone Boulevard, slants south at Brown University, and ends when it reaches the Seekonk River in Fox Point. Fox Point has been gentrified now, but when I was a girl it was a rundown neighborhood populated by recent immigrants from Portugal and the Cape Verde Islands. Triple-deckers crowded a Catholic family onto each floor—in the days when Catholics followed papal edicts about birth control. Poorly caulked windows rattled in the panes when the wind blew, and the smells of linguica sausage, fava beans, and kale wafted down back staircases. Hope Street ended there, stopping just short of the stinking Seekonk River, its waters bile green with pollution.

I learned to say, when people asked me where I lived, "Off of Hope." If they asked which side, I'd say, "The wrong side." That meant the west side, close to Camp Street, which was the heart of the East Side black ghetto.

My father took Jane, John, and me to register at our new school, Summit Avenue Elementary. In the auditorium we talked with the principal, Miss McGuinn, a woman whose bearing and dress conveyed the fact that she considered middle age to be the height of a woman's glory. She wore a purple dress that reached midcalf, and atop her bosom, which jutted forward like the prow of a ship bound to colonize far-off, heathen lands, was a fabric rose, a slightly paler shade of mauve than her dress. Her graying hair matched her dress, for it, too, had been tinted purple. Need I add that she had ramrod straight posture?

Miss McGuinn took one look at me and said, "We have a very fine school for handicapped children here in Providence."

"She's always gone to regular school," my father said.

"She'll have to climb stairs."

"She can climb stairs. The exercise is good for her."

Within a few days I learned that when Miss McGuinn entered our classroom the entire class was to rise to its feet—I was exempted from the requirement to rise—and intone in unison, "Good morning, Miss McGuinn." We were not to drone! We were to speak with enthusiasm! Every syllable of the word "en-thu-si-asm" was distinctly and separately enunciated. The students at the nearby parochial school greeted adults who entered the classroom in this way. Miss McGuinn made it clear that she regarded public schooling as a poor substitute for the education we might have had at the nearby Holy Name of Jesus School, from the Sisters of Notre Dame de Namur, with their starched coifs and wimples and wooden rulers ever at the ready for delivering a good hard swat to any of their charges who proved recalcitrant.

In Providence I was sometimes asked, "Are you Catholic or Jewish?" The word "Unitarian" required an explanation, so I took to saying "Protestant," although once one of my classmates responded "What's that?" "Sort of like Catholic, but without the pope," I fudged, as that was an explanation that seemed to make me less odd than other people.

Our house in Hamilton had ceilings so low that my Uncle Pete, six feet tall, had to stoop when he went through doorways. The kitchen floor sloped because the earth had settled underneath it in the century since it had been built. Upstairs, where my father had added on to the house so that we would each have our own bedroom, the windows he had built slanted at odd angles, and there were gaps between the baseboards and the plasterboard. Once Debby and I wrote "I hate Sandra" over and over again on scraps of paper and flung them into her bedroom through one of the holes my father had left in the wall.

Our new Victorian house, which we could afford because of its location on the wrong side of Hope and because most people then wanted split levels in the suburbs, had twelve rooms, a carriage house in the back, a magnificent stained-glass window, a formal front staircase with an elaborately carved bannister, eleven-foot ceilings, a living room with a row of dark polished beams running across the ceiling. The walls were thick and the doors solid hardwood.

The lofty ceilings in those enormous rooms made the house expensive to heat. Our first year there the furnace conked out in midwinter because we'd used up all the oil in the tank. When we'd signed up to become customers of DiPrete Oil, they'd sent us a potted philodendron with a gigantic red bow on it. The tanker truck returned and refilled the tank in our cellar, while my father groaned, "Now we know why they sent us that plant!" I watched his face, trying to gauge whether he meant this as a comment tinged with rueful irony or if he was really angry. I learned to dread the sight of the truck that delivered oil, the thick hose that snaked from it down into our basement, as it meant my father would be in a bad mood for days.

"Who turned the thermostat up?"

"If you're cold, put on a goddamn sweater."

"What the hell are you doing! Shut the door! You're letting the warm air out and the hot air in. Jesus Christ! I am not made of money."

"Do you know how much I have to pay for oil to heat this goddamn house? Me, I'm the one who's paying for it. It all comes out of my goddamn pocket."

When we came home from school in the afternoon, the house was cold and dark. My mother was usually gone because she was taking classes at Brown, getting a master's degree in teaching. The house's vast, high-ceilinged rooms seemed to contain great quantities of chilly emptiness. Sandra figured out that if she took an ice cube and held it against the thermostat, she could get the furnace to kick on without turning the thermostat up, and every day, when she got home, she got an ice cube out of the tray in the freezer and rubbed it against the thermostat until we heard the welcoming sound of the furnace chugging on and the radiators starting to hiss.

Things did not go well for my father at Brown. I know almost nothing of what happened there, beyond the fact that he did not receive the tenure he had expected. I have never known, and to this day do not know, which came first: Was it his accelerating craziness that made things fall apart for him at Brown, or did problems at his job send him spiraling more deeply into his madness? Although in many ways it was the central event of our family's life, it has never been spoken about beyond a few quickly tossed-off sentences.

My father's wild anger at Sandra, which had flared occasionally when we lived in Hamilton, now smoldered constantly in the background, occasionally turning into a conflagration that seemed as if it might consume us all. It might be set off by her getting a phone call, by the clothes that she wore; by the fact that, on a day she was home from school sick, she had answered the front door in her pajamas and bathrobe.

A year or so after we had moved to Providence, we all sat down at the dinner table. Without warning, without a word having been spoken, my father picked up his glass of water and flung the water in Sandra's face.

"I saw the way you looked at me."

She sat there with humiliation and confusion on her face, while water dripped from her hair, running down her face, mixing with her tears.

"Daddy," she protested. "I didn't look at you—"

"Shut up!"

"May I be excused, please?" Sandra said to my mother.

"No, you may not be excused," my father shouted.

Sandra lifted the napkin to her face, trying to sop up the water from her hair, her face, but the thin paper quickly became soaked and started to shred.

I fastened my eyes on my plate. I was scared to look at my father. I couldn't bear to look at Sandra. Around me our dinner rituals were going on as if nothing out of the ordinary had happened. My father asked my brother which piece of chicken he wanted, and my brother said, "The drumstick." The drumstick was set on the top plate of the stack of seven plates in front of my father, and then the plate was passed from Susan to me, from me to my mother, and the frozen peas that my mother had boiled and dabbed with a square of margarine were added to his plate, along with a couple of serving spoonfuls of instant mashed potatoes. Jane was next—my father gave her a thigh, and then we passed the plate along so my mother could serve her the vegetables. Then it was my turn. All the while Sandra sat with her hair dripping water onto her blouse, choking back tears.

I was watching the Beatles on television with my sister Jane. My father came into the room, and asked, his voice filled with a kind of false jollity it sometimes had after he'd had several drinks, "Are these the Beatniks?"

No sooner had Jane said, "Be quiet," than my father walloped her with a closed fist. His blow was so hard that it lifted her up from the couch and sent her flying backward across the room. She looked almost like a cartoon character who has just taken a punch, the way her head was flung back and her back arched from the force of the blow. Except this wasn't a cartoon. She wasn't the cat in the Tom and Jerry cartoons, who got blown up by a firecracker, had all his fur burned off, and then appeared in the next frame as if nothing had happened. This was my sister Jane, my flesh-and-blood sister, flying backward across the room.

While I can remember the incongruity of the sight—how it simultaneously made me think of a cartoon and was one of the scariest things I'd ever witnessed—I can't remember what happened afterward. Was the television turned off and were we sent to our rooms? Did I say anything to Jane afterward? Did I offer her sympathy? Did I hold her? Did I tell her I hated him, too? Or was I furious at her for having said "Be quiet," for not following the cardinal rule of our family: Don't upset him.

The next day my mother was giving me a ride somewhere, and I said, "Daddy shouldn't have hit Jane like that."

My mother glanced over at me briefly and said, "She told him to be quiet." Then she fixed her eyes on the road, fixed her hands on the steering wheel. "If I had known you felt that way, I wouldn't have given you a ride."

When I was twelve or thirteen, my sister Susan and I were in the den, arguing about what we were going to watch on television.

"Let's flip a coin," one or the other of us said, and we did.

I called heads, and the coin came up heads.

"I don't care," Susan said, and planted herself in front of the knob on the television.

"I won!" I yelled. "I won! This isn't fair!"

The next thing we knew, my father was standing in the doorway. "Cut it out," my father said, pointing his left index finger at me.

"We flipped a coin, and I won."

"Let your sister watch what she wants to watch."

"But, Dad, we flipped a coin, and I won."

"Be kind," my father said. "Be gentle. Give in." When he started this triumvirate of commands, he was maudlin. By the time he had gotten to the end of his list, he was in full rage. Was I foolish enough to protest again, "But, Dad—"? I don't remember. My memory goes blank until I am lying flat on my back on the couch in the living room, with my father's hands around my neck, choking off my air.

Although I have no actual memory, I can extrapolate, the way I did to create the mornings of my early childhood. My father must have said to me, "Come in the living room, so I can talk to you." When I see those words written on the page, they seem to have such workaday paternalism. He could say the word "you" and make it sound like a curse.

He would have sat me down on the couch and said, "The Bible teaches us to turn the other cheek." This is one of my father's most-often-used lines, despite the fact that he is an atheist, despite the fact of his own wild violence. I have learned to dread these words, as they often precede my being hit.

I can't imagine that I argued with him. Maybe I cowered, frightened, and in my cowering, my fear, my father saw himself reflected in my eyes. Maybe I did argue with him. Maybe it was the sight of my crippled body that filled him with rage, filling him with some atavistic revulsion and hate.

My father was wearing a suit, a necktie with a blue-and-red floral pattern. It flip-flopped back and forth as he battered my head up and down, up and down, on the arm of the sofa. Above us was the Breughel print of the *Peasants' Wedding Feast*; next to the couch a Danish modern lamp. A sharp pain cut into my windpipe as his thumbs pressed against it. I was gasping for air, unable to get it, just as I had gasped for air when the black ether mask was lowered over my face.

Would I survive this? I wasn't at all sure that I would. His face, distorted with rage, hovered above me as he squeezed, harder and harder. This would stop, I told myself. It would stop. I had gone through these chokings before, and he had always stopped himself in time. At least as far as I can remember now he always stopped before I passed out.

But then I have the voice of Jane telling me about an event I don't remember: an afternoon when she and my mother came home from shopping on a Saturday afternoon, and looked at each other, puzzled. What was that strange knocking noise coming from upstairs? It sounded like someone throwing furniture around. They went up the stairs and discovered my father, beating me so hard it sounded like thunder. My mother opened the door, grabbed me, got me out of the room, yelled to Jane and me, "Go! Run! Get out of the house! Go over to the Kiberds!" And stayed to face my father's rage alone. But I have absolutely no memory of that afternoon. And I always wonder what else I don't remember.

He wasn't stopping. Some force had him in its grip, as surely as I was in his grip, that wouldn't let him stop banging my head back and forth against the arm of the couch, wouldn't let him let go of my neck, to let up the pressure of his hands.

Was my face turning pale? Was it turning blue?

Usually I just lay there and took it, because I knew that doing anything else would only make him angrier. This time, I knew I had to do something. It was pure animal instinct, my heart pounding out its order: not *lub-dub, lub-dub,* but "LIVE-live, LIVE-live." I tried to move my hands up, to get them around his wrists, so I could pull his hands away from my neck. Futile, of course: He was so much stronger than me. I tried to scream, but no sound could get past his hands.

And then I managed to get out the words: "Mommy! Mommy! Help! Help!"

And then the next thing I remember, he was sitting on the couch, not choking me anymore, just yelling at me, "Why did you call her? This doesn't have anything to do with her." It was the voice of a three-year-old, in trouble with his own mother.

My mother stood in the doorway, in a triangle of light. "Don't upset your father," she said.

Then she told me to go to my room.

When I left the living room, I saw that the light had been turned off in the den, and none of the flickering pale light from the black-and-white television escaped from beneath the door. After all that, Susan wasn't even watching the program. I was furious at her. I had gone through all that, and she hadn't even really wanted to watch that program.

It was only years later I realized that she must have heard, even through the thick walls and doors, the sounds of what was happening in the living room, and slunk upstairs, sick with guilt.

What happened afterward? Did my father weep, as he sometimes did after these episodes? Did my mother comfort him? Did he have a drink? I am almost certain that he must have had a drink—not one of the two double martinis that he drank before dinner every night, but one of those drinks called a highball, a mix of whiskey and water, that he drank steadily throughout the evening—a single drink, freshened with more whiskey. Whiskey and gin, tamping down his rage but also loosening his inhibitions.

Did my mother come up to my bedroom and explain that my father was acting this way because he had quit smoking, warning me that quitting smoking was very difficult and so I must be especially careful not to upset him?

The morning after my father had choked me and banged my head against the arm of the sofa, I came down the stairs in my pajamas and bathrobe and walked through that room as if nothing had happened. I poured myself a cup of Maxwell House coffee from the electric percolator. My mother said, "Good morning," and I must have grunted back my muffled I-haven't-had-my-coffee-yet "Good morning," and then headed back to my bedroom, carrying the mug carefully so it didn't slosh out as my body swayed from side to side, walking again through the living room.

Sometimes, on Saturday nights, my parents would have people over. They would offer their guests drinks—highballs, martinis, maybe even a sloe gin fizz. Sometimes at these parties, when some of the guests were smoking cigarettes and my father longed for one, he would turn to my mother and say, "Mary El, smoke a cigarette."

And my mother would dutifully light up a cigarette and smoke it.

The U.S. surgeon general had recently come out with a report that fully fleshed out the hazards of smoking, and the newspapers were filled with stories about people quitting smoking, and tips on how to stop.

I hated the surgeon general, and I hated his report.

I went to the Cumberland Farms store on Camp Street and said, "A pack of Camels," and pushed a dime, a nickel, and a pile of pennies across the counter. The man behind the counter picked out thirty-one cents and slid the rest of the pennies back toward me. My homeroom teacher, Mr. Marino, on whom I had a crush, smoked Camels. A pack was always visible through the thin cloth of his white polyester shirts.

Before I climbed up the rickety stairs to the second floor of the carriage house, I picked up a bottle of mouthwash from the medicine cabinet in the bathroom and shoved it into my jacket pocket. The carriage house was filled with the detritus of nearly a century—a broken leather harness, cans of half-used paint, and abandoned cardboard boxes and wooden boxes with hinged lids. When we had first moved to Providence, we'd come upon them and unfold lids which hadn't been moved in decades, half believing, as in children's stories, that within we'd find some secret treasures—old-fashioned dresses, mysterious letters, perhaps a pocket watch with a strange inscription that would lead us on a search. Instead we'd discovered piles of rusty hardware, panes of glass.

Upstairs in the musty carriage house, repeating the gesture I had seen my father perform so often, I grabbed the red cellophane tail on my pack of cigarettes and pulled. The noise the cellophane packaging made as I crumpled it was familiar. I thrust it into my pocket—it was now evidence that must be disposed of. I peeled back the silver paper, and tapped the pack against my hand with a debonair flick of my wrist, but three or four cigarettes didn't pop free of the pack as they did on cigarette commercials. Instead I had to reach in and grab one between my thumb and forefinger, yank it free.

"I smoke," I said to myself. I imagined myself as a character on a TV show or in a movie. The male lead would ask me, as he proffered a pack of cigarettes, "Do you smoke?" and I would say, in a sultry voice, "Thank you," as I leaned forward and took a cigarette from his pack. He would light my cigarette, and I would slowly, sexily, draw smoke deeply into my lungs. Our eyes would meet.

I lit the cigarette and took a first initial puff, and began to cough.

After a few puffs of the cigarette I felt dizzier than when I used to twirl myself around and around on the swing in the front yard of the house in Hamilton. My head ached, as if my brain had turned into a bass drum a drummer was hitting over and over again with an enormous mallet.

My father was lying on the floor of the front hallway, crying out, moaning, the way a child having a temper tantrum will when they can't get themselves to cry but want everyone around to know how upset they are. "She *hit* me."

I was standing on the stairs, watching him. Had I heard a strange noise and come down from my bedroom to see what was going on? Or did I just happen to be going up or down the stairs when he came through the door from the living room and flung himself down onto the floor?

He was kicking his legs back and forth and crying out, "She hit me. She hit me right in the solar plexus. It hurts! Oh, it hurts!"

I had experienced enough physical pain that I could tell my father was not in the kind of pain that sends you onto the floor, clutching at yourself and groaning.

He folded his arms across his midsection, bent himself double. "Right in the solar plexus! She hit me! Oh, it hurts, it hurts, it hurts!"

I tried to imagine what had happened on the other side of the door. To imagine my mother balling her hand into a fist and slugging my father in the gut. And, despite all my mother's gentleness, I could see her doing this. I could imagine her sweet demeanor finally breaking down, a cold anger settling over her the way it sometimes did, her lips forming a thin line. But I knew he must have been hitting her first, maybe even choking her. I was glad she had hit him back, finally.

This is the man who is the head of our house. This man, lying on the floor, crying and carrying on like a two-year-old having a temper tantrum.

I told Jane, "Mom hit Dad."

"No, she didn't."

"She did. He was lying on the floor, crying."

"She didn't," Jane almost shouted at me. "She didn't hit him."

My mother came down to breakfast with a black eye. She said that my father was turning over in the night and hit her eye with his elbow.

My grades plummeted. I flunked a spelling test. The part of my psyche that was sending a distress signal to the world must have had to be working overtime in order for me to flunk a spelling test—for the past few years, I'd been the kid on the edge of the playground with my nose in a book. Miss Wood, the teacher, had me come to redo the quiz after the end of the school day. I sat in the classroom, surrounded by twenty-nine empty wooden desks and seats. The air was plangent with the smells of chalk dust and adolescent sweat. Outside, beyond the closed door of Room 212, the occasional shouts of other kids—on their way to football practice or just released from detention—ricocheted off the walls.

While I was writing the words she was dictating to me, "Plummet. The stones *plummet* to the earth. Plummet. . . . Rhinoceros. The *rhinoceros* bathed in the watering hole. Rhinoceros . . . ," tears started to well in my eyes. I had no idea what I was crying about. I wasn't even aware of being sad. I knew only that I was crying, and felt sheepish for doing so. I bent my head down, letting my long hair fall like a curtain around my face, wiped my eyes with my fingers, and hoped Miss Wood wouldn't notice.

"Rhythm. The dancers swayed in time to the *rhythm* of the music. Rhythm."

A tear fell from my eye, landed on the thin blue-lined sheet of paper on which we wrote our spelling quizzes, splotching the ink. I moved my elbow quickly, in an attempt to hide the blotch.

But she had seen, and leaned over, took the test away from me, scrawled "100" on the top of it, and asked me "What's the matter?"

"I don't know," I managed to say.

"Everything okay with your friends?"

I nodded.

"What about at home?"

In place of an answer, I started to cry harder. Finally I managed to say, "My dad's too strict."

She rubbed her hand on my shoulder. "You know, if they tell you you can't do something, and you really want to do it—just go ahead. What's your father going to do? He's not going to hit you," she said.

She is so certain that such a thing could never happen, and I cannot begin to find the words to tell her that it has gone so much further than that.

———

Beyond spankings I don't think John and Susan were ever hit. John because he was a boy, and Susan because she was the "good daughter." Although even being good wasn't a lot of protection in our family. When she was a junior in high school, Susan was not only a straight-A student, she also held down a forty-hour-a-week job. And not just any job. She'd started out volunteering at the local theater company, Trinity, and had been so good that they'd hired her to paint sets and run lights. Trinity was just beginning to build the national reputation it has today, and didn't yet have a real theater of its own; it was housed in the basement of a church on the far side of downtown, without any place for those who worked on sets to clean up at the end of their shifts. When a new play was in rehearsal and Susan was working on sets, she'd ride the bus home in the paint-splattered clothes. She'd walk in the door and my father would start yelling, "I will not have a daughter of mine going around looking like that."

"Daddy, we were painting sets."

"You're *my* daughter. People see you on the bus, and they know you're *my* daughter."

"Daddy, I can't put my school clothes back on; they'll get paint all over them." This argument happened time after time. At the time it didn't seem that disturbing to me—after all, it was just yelling, it never went any further than that. But when I was the mother of an adolescent, I thought if I had a teenager like Susan, I'd wonder what I had done right in a previous life, I'd get down on my knees and thank the God I didn't believe in.

I only remember Jane getting that one out-of-control wallop, and my father's anger at Sandra was almost always verbal. I was the one who bore the brunt of his physical rage. Sometimes when I tell people this, they think he went after me because I was the weakest one, but I don't think that had anything to do with it. We were all scared of him, scared to fight back or even to resist. His anger toward me was physical, rage at that body of mine that persisted, despite all the promises that had been made to us, despite all that had been done for it, despite all that had been done to it, in remaining crippled. His daughter's body—and for him, the operative word in that phrase was "his"—which walked up and down Hope Street leaning heavily on its crutches, drawing stares, some curious, some sympathetic. Out there for all the world to see, the physical manifestation of the inner state of our family—broken, bent, crippled, wrong.

CRIPPLING GENDER

I

As a disabled girl I was allowed to have dreams and ambitions that were denied to nearly all other girls in the 1950s. When we went around the room in Miss Huggins's fifth-grade class and said what we wanted to be when we grew up, the boys said, "farmer" and "fire-fighter," "jet pilot," "astronaut," and all the other girls in the class said either "nurse" or "teacher." I don't even remember what I said at that point—archaeologist? doctor? writer?—because I was so busy being incensed and perplexed at the other girls, so busy thinking, What is the *matter* with them? and maybe feeling saddened, too, at the way their dreams had already been stunted. (How the world has changed and not changed—when my son was in elementary school, all the girls in his fifth-grade class wanted to be either veterinarians or pediatricians.) When you had polio it didn't matter if you were a boy or a girl: You were always being told about President Roosevelt. You were expected to be smart, to be accomplished, to make something of your life, maybe even grow up to be president.

Not surprisingly polio affected males and females differently. Daniel Wilson, who himself had polio, has written of how polio "crippled manhood," forcing boys and men consciously to make or remake their masculine selves. He detailed the ideal of masculinity in the 1940s and 1950s that was marked by actively participating in sports, exhibiting physical strength, being sexually attractive to women, earning a living and supporting one's family financially, and serving in the military. Since males who had polio were shut out from many of these activities, their masculinity became a conundrum.

One of the "dangers" for males who had polio was that the disease would make them weak and effeminate—in the parlance of the day, "sissies." Wilson points out that this "anxiety about sissies was caught up in the post–World War II fears about communism and homosexuality. Americans believed that men needed to be strong, resilient, masculine if the nation was to resist the global spread of communism." Communism itself was often characterized as a disease—it spread, like a cancer or an epidemic. Wilson continues, "Boys who were sissies were thought to be especially susceptible to homosexuality . . . and, as homosexuals, potential pawns of communists." The threat went beyond the fact that the nation's "strength depended upon the ability of strong manly men to stand up against communist threats"; a homosexual was easy prey for Communists who might uncover his predilections and blackmail him into betraying his country.

Often these concerns about the threats polio posed to normal masculinity were covert and coded, but sometimes this fear was made explicit. One boy who had had polio overheard his grandmother telling his father that she had read "most of the polio victims will grow up being homosexual because very few of the opposite sex will want to be seen with a cripple. The polio victim will be forced into a life of solitude or homosexuality." One should remember that the stereotype of the homosexual in those days was not that of a latte drinker with an expensive haircut and a well-tailored suit, urbane and witty, lending his suave eye to the beleaguered straight guy, taking part each June in a gay pride march, getting married to his longtime partner in a ceremony at San Francisco's city hall, but of a man whose fear of having his terrible secret unmasked made him an ever-wary social misfit. He was at home only in shadowy alleys, sleazy movie theaters, the stalls of public men's rooms.

These assumptions did not just circulate idly through the national conversation. In the late 1940s and 1950s, gay baiting was nearly as common as Red baiting, and like the anti-Communist witch hunts also destroyed careers and forced those who "confessed their guilt" to name others. That these ruthless investigations seeking to uncover homosexuality among government employees and "subversives" were carried out by the FBI, then headed by closeted homosexual J. Edgar Hoover, is another sad irony of history.

Both women and men who had had polio faced overwhelming job discrimination. For men such discrimination not only threatened them financially and in terms of status but attacked their masculine identity. Larry Alexander wrote, "When I get to the point where I can make a living . . . I'll be a complete man again." In the 1930s, when Sylvia Flexer Bassoff found that she couldn't get a job "not because there was a Depression," she recounted years later, but "because I was handicapped," the experience, while profoundly discouraging, does not seem to have threatened her identity as a female. But, on the other hand, if her sense of herself as a woman had been wounded by polio, achieving employment did not restore it.

Leonard Kriegel, disabled—he would say crippled—by polio at the age of eleven, believed "you were better off struggling with the effects of disease as a man than as a woman," since battling the disease's aftereffects involved being "tough, aggressive, and decisive." An opposite argument could be made. The toughness and sense of drive one was expected to exhibit as one struggled to become as "normal" as possible in the wake of polio provided a corrective to the passivity and weakness expected of girls, while it exaggerated male traits.

Certainly Kriegel has been the most prolific—and engaging—writer on the subject of manhood in the wake of polio. In essays and memoirs he has returned again and again to his experience of polio and its effect on his masculine identity, often mulling over the crucial weeks and months when he was wrenched away from being a working-class son of immigrants on New York's Lower East Side—unexceptional in his dreams that sandlot baseball would lead to a career in the big leagues; perhaps slightly ashamed of his immigrant parents, his shame tempered by the fact that nearly all his friends had parents who spoke English with the same Yiddish inflection, who seemed never to be quite at home in this strange America; just starting on the path from boyhood to manhood. Polio rocketed Kriegel out of his familiar world, like the tornado that whirled Dorothy out of Kansas, first to an acute-care hospital and then to the New York State Reconstruction Home. The shift was far more than geographic: He was also tumbled into a world where maleness was no longer a sure and steady anchor.

Often in his writing Kriegel assumes the pose of a curmudgeon, yearning for a simpler day, weighing in against all that is newfangled: cultural relativism, virtual reality, current ignorance of Greek myth, the drumbanging psuedomasculinity of Robert Bly, "politically correct" language. Kriegel defiantly uses the word "cripple" to describe himself. The word "cripple" has always been a slur; in the last few decades that easy pejorative no longer seems socially acceptable. Beyond that, it is beginning to have an antiquated air, rather like describing someone as "feeble-minded." A derivative of "cripple," "crip" is used within the disabled community, a code word that marks you as being part of the group, a word only insiders are allowed to use. Kriegel does not use the word "crip" to indicate his brotherhood with other disabled people, who seem markedly lacking from his life once he has left the hospital behind. He uses the word "cripple" because he wants to set himself apart from the speakers of euphemism. "Cripple." Not "mobility-impaired," "disabled," "orthopedic." Kriegel wants to let us know he is no lily-livered bureaucrat who pushes such language around on his desk. He is the kind of man who can take on a word like "cripple."

The opening essay in his book *Flying Solo: Reimagining Manhood, Courage, and Loss* opens with Kriegel and another boy, also recovering from polio, who have just been lifted from a pool of hot water. They lie near each other, awaiting another immersion, "passive in exhaustion," languorous, enervated. "In a few minutes, we would each feel that hot water lapping our necks, shriveling world and body with the loss and pain being sweated out of us."

The essay is titled "Being Done." The phrase is one the long-term boys—"who swaggered in their wheelchairs like Bogarts and Cagneys"—used with the newcomers. Polio had "done" you, they said. You were done, a ready-to-come-out-of-the-oven Thanksgiving turkey or Shabbos chicken. Your goose was cooked. To strip away all the turns of phrase, the verbal niceties, to put it in plain and simple English: You were fucked. Yes, the disease had entered these boys. And now this disease had split them open, it had gone more deeply into them than they could ever have gone into a woman, it had entered into the very cells of their bodies. It had made them weak, weak but not flaccid. Kriegel's muscles had been contracted, leaving him "stiff as a newly varnished board." And he lay on his back, waiting to be dipped again in hot water, which would embrace him, soothing away pain but also cooking his body into limpness.

Kriegel, flat on his back, had been forced to take the supine position that women were supposed to assume in sex, the same position as when "laid up" with illness. Real men stood up, they walked, they ran, they strode, they marched, they swaggered. No doubt on that very day—early

September 1944—men were tromping in platoons and brigades through muddy fields in France; their feet were slapping against the steps of a steel staircase as they raced to man battle stations on ships in the Pacific; if they drifted at all, they were drifting on currents of air, having parachuted out of a burning plane or been dropped behind enemy lines to meet up with a Resistance unit in France or Albania. "Motion and manhood," Kriegel writes elsewhere. "A simple equation."

These were men—or so it must have seemed to Kriegel—for whom manhood was never a question. It was as natural as having two legs that moved forward without any conscious thought at all.

"Yet I cannot afford," Kriegel remembers decades later, "to recognize what really disturbs me." The memory returns to him, he says, as if it were "a dirty little secret." Shame seeps through the text. "Will I ever be a man among men?" The virus has also taken from him his faith in the steady ground of masculinity. Disability teaches us lessons, whether we want to learn them or not. What had seemed since the day he was born— "It's a boy!"—to be an incontrovertible statement has become one filled with questions. An earthquake had revealed that the land on which he had constructed his psychic house, which he had assumed to be bedrock, was in fact silt, leaving his once-solid state of manliness a pile of rubble.

Confronting such ruins, one can choose either to rebuild—or to strike out for new territory. Kriegel determined that he would not decamp, not find some other answer to this puzzle that his manhood had suddenly become. He would reconstruct himself as a man. He would do this by making polio his adversary.

What does it mean to make a disease one's enemy? It is an idea so deeply embedded in our culture that it seems natural. The patient sitting in the doctor's office, his head bent low under the weight of the news he has just received, says, "I'm going to fight it, Doc." The doctor, walking with solemn footsteps toward the expectant family, anxious in the waiting room, slowly pulls the stethoscope from around his neck and, after having cast his eyes briefly downward, breaks the news by saying: "He was a real fighter. . . ." The death notice reads, "After a long battle with cancer . . ." Kriegel determined that he would be the boxer who has had the living daylights beaten out of him, punch-drunk, fated to be defeated, but not giving up. On the mat, hearing the ref's count above him, he will stagger to his feet and make one last bold foray against his opponent.

In another of his books Kriegel writes of having adopted Hemingway not as a literary mentor but as a "nurse." Hemingway's hypermasculinity—his ostentatious big-game hunting and fishing, the toughness of his prose, his displays of raw physical courage—provide Kriegel a way of remaking his masculinity:

> I remember, soon after I began to read Hemingway, walking mile after mile with my crutches literally eating into the pits of my shoulders, thinking that I was somehow going to gain the approval of a man who did not even know of my existence and who would, no doubt, have been puzzled if not openly appalled at the role which I insisted he accept.

Polio was, in Kriegel's mind, "personified as a living, malevolent being." Although it would no doubt embarrass him to admit it, his attitude bears more than a passing resemblance to that of the late-nineteenth-century disabled poet, William Ernest Henley, who authored that favorite of inspirational speakers and givers of commencement addresses, *Invictus*:

> My head is bloody, but unbowed.
> . . . I am the master of my fate:
> I am the captain of my soul.

Every man performs his masculinity, but the disabled man must become conscious of doing so. Kriegel even went so far as to make a list of the things that he had to accomplish and achieve in order to regain his lost manhood. Passing from boyhood to manhood cannot be something that happens, seemingly without effort, through the passage of time. It must be envisioned, planned for, pursued with purpose.

How do disabled women exist in his mind? Have we taken up residence in some forgotten back room, where the air has grown musty from its door having rarely been opened; there perhaps we lounge, à la Elizabeth Barrett Browning, on a dusty settee, thin, pale, and growing every day paler. In Kriegel's writings we become mere outlines, "an olive-skinned girl" with whom he will "lock chairs . . . behind the red-brick laundry, fumbling away at her as I try to forget dead legs in the soft feel of flesh beneath her gray wool sweater."

But other than that, disabled women are invisible in all his texts, and he can see hypermasculinity as the only response to disability.

II

But polio didn't disrupt gender only for those who had the disease. Let us return to that emblematic figure, our forthright Australian, Sister Kenny—or "Sister Ken" as she was sometimes called.

The year was 1946. New York's Times Square. A movie premiere. Limousines, a red carpet, policemen holding back the adoring crowds. Lights danced around the movie marquee of the RKO Palace. The throng was so thick that the limousines couldn't get to the front of the theater, and the guests, coming from the preparty, were dropped off at some distance and then ushered by policemen through the jostling crowd. The guest of honor, arrayed in white—a white sequined dress, pearls, white gloves—arrived in a limousine, although she demonstrated a democratic touch by riding in front with the driver. A platform had been set up in front of the theater so she could say a few words to those assembled. As she was finishing her brief thanks, the press of bodies against a barrier caused it to give way, the crowd surged against the temporary platform, which swayed precariously, and strong hands reached up to grab and steady the woman on the platform, rescuing her from the surging weight of adulation.

The woman the crowd had been straining toward wasn't Lana Turner or Rita Hayworth. In fact, she was the distinct opposite of a 1940s glamour girl: an imposing, broad-shouldered woman who spoke not in a sex-kittenish purr but with a down-to-earth Australian twang. And she wasn't the star of the movie, but its subject. Rosalind Russell, who played the lead in *Sister Kenny*, had stayed away, wanting her friend to get the evening's glory.

Order restored, Elizabeth Kenny made her way along the red carpet. Occasionally she turned and smiled at those held back behind the barricades, with a look that seemed to say, *Isn't it funny, all this hoopla over me!* No doubt more than one woman in the crowd could imagine herself and the object of her admiration sitting down together at a kitchen table, sharing a cup of coffee and swapping stories: The woman they had gathered to see had that mix of grandeur and unpretentiousness Americans expect from our celebrities.

Just a year and a half previously, Times Square wouldn't have been illuminated as it was that night. Wartime authorities had ordered that the neon signs and rows of flashing incandescent lights above theaters, movie palaces, and dance halls be dimmed, not just to save electricity but because they were so bright they silhouetted ships offshore, making them more vulnerable to attack by German U-boats. But still, despite the military restrictions, people had packed into Times Square—mainly women, alone and in groups, although there were sometimes also soldiers and sailors on leave. They emerged out of the darkness into patches of soft light glowing from the interiors of restaurants and the lobbies of theaters; the eerie near-darkness seeming to enhance the sense of drama and camaraderie.

Now that the war was over, lights blazed again in marquees and signs, theaters, and cinemas, and in advertisements for Gillette razor blades, Buitoni spaghetti, Planters peanuts: postwar consumerism coming into its own. Advertisements and magazine stories, which just a few years before had urged women to join the workforce, now encouraged women to return to their homes, and promised postwar technological abundance. Surely some of the women in the crowd who gathered to pay tribute to Sister Elizabeth Kenny yearned to have, in some small part, a life like hers. A life submerged in a larger cause, as perhaps theirs had been during the war; one in which feminine giving produced not passivity but an almost bulldog sense of assertion—and no small amount of glory.

After the movie of her life was released, she became so famous that when she entered New York nightclubs, the emcee would announce her presence: "Ladies and gentlemen! Will you please join me in welcoming to our midst a great, great lady, Sister Elizabeth Kenny!" The spotlight would rake across the crowd until it came to rest on her, she would stand up and bow her head a bit, stretch forth her magical hands. When the applause died down, the band leader would say, "And now in Sister Kenny's honor, we will be playing her favorite song, 'Danny Boy,'" and as the band struck up the sentimental tune, her eyes would well with tears, as they always did when she heard this song.

Some people—notably the publicists at RKO—claimed she loved this song because there was a man named Dan she'd left behind in Australia—abandoned him so she could purpose "the work"; although others said, "Sister Ken! A beau! That's a good one!"

In Victor Cohn's biography of Kenny—a book that combines, in equal measure, frankness about and empathy for its subject—he tells of her romances. In her late twenties "she was keeping company, it was said, or thought she was, some insist," with Reg McAllister, a chemist—or pharmacist, in American English—who lived near her cousin, Minnie Moore Bell. Minnie Bell said flatly that there was "never any romance" between Elizabeth and Reg, although Cohn was told by another informant that the two of them were once caught by Elizabeth's grandmother "spooning and paloodling" in the kitchen.

Whatever "spooning and paloodling" may have involved, her brief relationship with Reg did not make it into her autobiography; a story about a romance with a man she called "Dan" did. Describing her last encounter with him, at the races that were the big event of the year, with people gathered from all across the countryside: "Twice during the past month he had been stern with me. I must give up this nursing nonsense if I were to take the place for which my Creator had ordained me."

But just as they were about to step into Dan's buggy, a boy rode up on horseback with the news that his mother was in premature labor and needed Nurse Kenny at once. Dan frowned at the news that she must go to the mother's aid. " 'You'll have to decide now,' Dan flared, 'whether you are to be married to me or to your vocation.' " A few minutes later, running up the stairs to change into her nurse's uniform, Elizabeth heard "the wheels of Dan's buggy grind as though in swift rage out of the driveway."

However, according to Victor Cohn, when the autobiography was published "some of Sister Kenny's former neighbors voiced doubt about Dan's existence. Her sisters were assuring yet vague on the subject, and none had ever met him. In her later years, she herself at times said conflicting things." One informant remembered her during her adolescence as someone who didn't "take part in our ordinary enjoyments, balls, dances and that sort of thing. She was what I would say more of the masculine type, in her usual manner—in make up [sic] and body build rather more like a man than a woman." When she served as a nurse in the Australian Army during World War I, she was known by the nickname "Ken."

Photographs of her as a young woman show an attractive, even beautiful woman; in fact, she was the one who often seemed to want little truck with romance. Once, on one of the hospital ships on which she worked that carried wounded soldiers back home to Australia during World War I, an admirer tried to woo her by saying, "Ah, those beautiful black eyes of yours with the faraway look, from gazing over the sea." She came back with: "Yes, like two burned holes in a blanket." And when the film of her life played up her supposed romance, she thundered: "Get them on the phone! I will not have them making me a cheap little pantry girl."

On more than one occasion Kenny said, "Men! I don't want anything to do with them." And: "I won't let any man boss me." Screenwriter Mary McCarthy (not to be confused with the eponymous author famous for writing *The Group* and feuding with Lillian Hellman) once asked her, "What do you hate the most?" Kenny, "like a Gatling gun," shot back: "[Going] to teas with a lot of fat, overdressed, over-bejewelled women who've never done one honest day's work." The statement combines pride in herself at being a member of the class of people who knew what it meant to do a hard day's work, along with contempt for the traditional female role. (One could also point out that there was a similarity between Kenny herself and those she hated: She herself was a large woman given to ornate dressing.) Was Kenny a lesbian? The possibility is hinted at, although never openly stated, in Cohn's biography; perhaps a current biography of Kenny, being written by Naomi Rogers, will address the question more openly.

Kenny was such a powerful presence that even after her death patients at the Kenny Institute in Minneapolis were told, during their physical therapy sessions, "Sister Kenny would not be proud of you," or, alternatively, "Good for you! Sister Kenny would be happy." Larry Kohout, who underwent polio rehabilitation there as a child, recalls "puffing up like a balloon" with pride on receiving the second comment.

In her native Australia she was regarded by many in the medical profession as a few steps removed from a quack. In the United States in the 1940s and 1950s, she was credited with almost miraculous healing powers. In the 1970s, when the feminist movement was searching for heroines, her image was resurrected as a woman healer who'd been maligned by the male-dominated medical profession. More recently she's been painted by some of her former patients as an abuser whose treatments were little more than medically sanctioned torture.

Elizabeth Kenny's autobiography paints a vivid portrait of herself as a tomboyish hoyden—roaming the bush, breaking horses, acting as physical trainer to her weakly brother. The years following girlhood are far less keenly drawn. It is not hard to infer that as adulthood approached, while her brothers saw their horizons widening, hers were narrowing. Employment opportunities open to her as a rural woman with scant formal education were few indeed. Womanhood was leading her into a dark tunnel from which she could see no way out.

Toward the end of the twentieth century, feminist author Miriam Dixson wrote that to be an Australian woman is to know one is expected: "to be tip-toe, dull, dolly-bird, blank-faced, 'don't crowd me love, I've got my mates.'" Dixson traced the formation of this attitude to the early days of white settlement in Australia, when the colony was populated mostly by convicts. The convicts were overwhelmingly male; and the society they built tended to exclude women from decision making and power, emphasizing women's service to men, and to forming powerful homosocial bonds. Australia has been described not so much as a patriarchal society as a fratriarchal one, where power is exercised by men acting in the roles of brothers rather than of fathers. That these attitudes long persisted in Australia can be illustrated by a few salient facts: In 1974 the Australian National University did not have a single woman professor. In that same year one of the few women ever to win a seat in the House of Representatives found herself asked to pose for newspaper photographs hanging her laundry on the line and preparing food in her kitchen.

Small wonder that a tough, independent-minded woman like Elizabeth Kenny would feel her life closing in on her as she attained her majority, and would find the question of her vocation a perplexing one. She sojourned with relatives, assisting them in their household duties—although showing far more interest in caring for children than in dusting and scrubbing. As she approached thirty, she seemed on her way to becoming a spinsterish eccentric who drove a cart with onions and potatoes and barley into the Queensland market.

Shortly before shooting on *Sister Kenny* began, the story got into the papers that Kenny had received a telegram from a firm of solicitors by the name of Craik and Gallager in Red Raven, New South Wales, Australia: "Daniel Lewellyn Montgomery passed away at his home November first. Desired this message to be sent to you. 'Here in the silent hills you loved so well I wait for thee.' Accept the sympathy of Craik and Gallager, Attorneys." (A Western Union blank with the notation COPY-CABLE and this message appears in Kenny's personal correspondence file at the Kenny Institute in Minnesota.) There is, however, no place named Red Raven in New South Wales, nor is there any record of a firm called Craik and Gallager. The telegram seems to have been a publicity stunt on the part of RKO.

Whatever Kenny's personal romantic life may have been, it is clear that studio executives knew that a movie in which a discussion of anterior horn cells, paralysis, spasm, alienation, and muscle reeducation needed some livening up, and romance.

And yet the romantic interest they created for Elizabeth Kenny—a military officer named Kevin Connors—was hardly a traditional one. True enough, at first sight Kevin Connors is conventionally masculine. Played by the square-jawed and square-shouldered Dean Jagger, he's an army officer, tall, resolute. But the role he plays is a feminized one. Kevin waits, yearning for what he cannot have. Even before the film audience sees him, we hear Kenny say that Captain Connors's supposed heroism—his fighting for the motherland in India—in fact consisted of his "sitting around on a small, bare hill in Afghanistan."

The story line that runs throughout the romantic subplot of the film is Kevin's attempt to get Elizabeth to tear herself away from her patients and pay attention to him. In one series of scenes he calls repeatedly after her "Liz!" while she rushes from one doctor's office to another discussing infantile paralysis and muscle reeducation. She puts off their wedding repeatedly. At one point he says, "My only chance of getting any attention from you is to get sick myself."

In fact, their most impassioned scene does occur when Kevin has been wounded in World War I. In the film—as in life—Kenny worked as a military nurse during the war. In the movie version, Kevin has been wounded, and as he lies flat on his back on a hospital bed, Kenny almost throws herself on top of him. Their encounter in this situation has not been by chance. It took will and determination—and once again, Kenny was the active one: She reveals to Kevin that she arranged to have them both transferred so they could be together. "Ah, Liz," gushes Kevin, "if I only had your brains."

It is not only in the romance plot that conventional sex roles are reversed. One of the crucial scenes of the film is between a child "crippled by the medical profession" and one of Sister Kenny's "miracles." The cripple is male; the healthy child is female. The girl—a bare-chested nymph (having just been examined by a doctor, she has removed her dress and is wearing nothing but her bloomers)—dances and turns cartwheels around the boy, who has braces on his legs and uses crutches. In a further violation of gender norms, the healthy girl is lovingly reprimanded by Sister Kenny, "Dory, look at those knees, you've got them all dirty. . . . Those hands aren't too clean either." It is the boy who is confined—we see him having been fetched from a room full of disabled children within a hospital—and when he leaves the scene, it is to be returned to that interior space. Dory's dirty hands and knees link her to an outdoor world of rough-and-tumble playfulness.

Another key scene in the film is a confrontation between Dr. Brack and Sister Kenny during "grand rounds"—a medical ritual in which one doctor lectures to other doctors and medical students. The setting is an amphitheater: The audience rises above Dr. Brack—previously encountered in the film as a polio expert—and a polio patient, a teenage boy naked save for a white loincloth.

The scene suggests a number of iconic paintings set in clinics. Among the best known of these are two by the nineteenth-century American painter Thomas Eakins. In one of his paintings, *The Gross Clinic* (the name is derived from the name of the physician, not as a description of what goes on there) the upper two-thirds of the painting is in shadow. The figures who loom above Dr. Gross—seated physicians, looking down on the drama unfolding beneath them—are barely discernible. A solitary female figure appears in this painting—as does a solitary female figure in another, similar Eakins painting, *The Agnew Clinic*. In *The Gross Clinic* the woman has not only averted her head from the proceedings but covers her eyes with her arm as well. Her hands claw the air. Clearly she is a figure of distress; standing in stark contrast to the rationality and detachment of the men who surround her. Who is she? Perhaps someone meant to assist in the surgery? But why then does she seem disturbed by and unaccustomed to the events that are unfolding? A relative of the patient, maybe? But why then has she been permitted into the operating theater? The viewer's inability to "get a reading" on her only increases her mystery and air of the irrational. (In *The Agnew Clinic* the female figure is less fraught but clearly subordinate: She wears a uniform, one that suggests simultaneously that of a nurse and a maid. She stands with a tray held impassively in front of her—containing not a tea service but the instruments the good doctor will need.) Eakins did not create these paintings sui generis; they draw on a long tradition of similar medical paintings featuring an almost theatrical setting.

In *Sister Kenny* we have the same ranks of tiered seats rising above an illuminated male figure who commands center stage. We have the same figure of the patient, lying pale and mute upon the table. The audience intent on Dr. Brack is all male, save for three silent women—grouped together, too matronly to suggest the Graces, they might be the Fates or the Furies: The white caps perched atop their coifs show them to be nurses. While the patient lies, constrained in splints, displayed before the watching medical audience, Dr. Brack lectures about the body before him: "This boy was brought here immediately, and I advised total immobilization."

And then Kenny enters the amphitheater, interrupting not just the lecture but the expected power relations between male and female, doctor and nurse. (Outside the world of the Hollywood film she seemed to do this as well. On physician Herbert Levine's first meeting with Kenny he found himself "caught . . . off guard by her brusqueness and directness . . . so stunned I could merely answer, 'Yes, ma'am' like a disobedient child.")

The film's Dr. Brack, however, responds to Kenny's sharpness not with obsequiousness but with unctuousness; Kenny is brash and abrasive—and so persistent that she forces Brack to give her an audience. The two of them parry back and forth. Kenny explains her theory of polio, including the terms "spasm" and "alienation." Dr. Brack responds: "Alienation—you'll find that word in the divorce court—these are not scientific words. They're gibberish—you've invented them." Defending immobilization, Dr. Brack says, "I can show you patients whose bodies are perfectly straight." To which Kenny responds, "Straight and rigid. There are thousands lying out in graveyards who have just as much chance of recovering the use of their legs." She later continues, "Your fathers bled their patients for everything from a fever to a cold. Do you do it anymore? Harvey changed a few ideas. So did Pasteur. I wish Pasteur were here." Dr. Brack responds, "So do I, Miss Kenny. He had a cure for hydrophobia."

What I am most struck by, though, is the way the patient remains silent throughout this encounter. The battle is fought over him; he remains motionless, passive, mute. Kenny has escaped from her subordination by challenging Brack; the patient now occupies the feminized role.

Memories of their scantily clad bodies being displayed in medical settings occur over and over again in the narratives of polio survivors. Richard Owen was examined by Sister Kenny in Indiana in the early 1940s, when he was a teenager. Kenny's visit to Indiana was a big event, and there were newspaper reporters and photographers on hand. Owen, who was wearing only a tiny loincloth, was terrified when a photographer from a local newspaper snapped a picture of him nearly naked. Was it going to appear in the local paper? Much to his relief, it didn't.

As a teenager Charles Mee had been operated on by a man who had the reputation of being a great and renowned surgeon. Although Mee lied about the results to his parents, who had been enthusiastic about the surgery, he acknowledged to himself that it had been "completely useless." The doctor who had performed it was proud of what he had done and often summoned Mee so that the results of his handiwork could be showed off to visiting physicians:

> I would arrive early, strip, and put on a little loincloth, like a diaper. This in itself was a disagreeable experience. I was, in any case, an embarrassable adolescent boy. But to be reduced to an object, as these days, finally, everyone knows, is profoundly diminishing. In fact, I was reduced to something even less than an object: I was a specimen." Mee would then be brought out on stage "like the elephant man."

With a wooden pointer the great doctor would go over the surgery he had done, using Mee's body as a pedagogical aid. Mee would be asked if he had been able to walk better after the surgery, and he would dutifully lie and say that yes, he could now walk better. Finally Mee figured out that if he told the truth, it would be the end of these visits. So the next time he was asked the question, he responded honestly, " 'No, I don't think it has made any difference at all, really; maybe I'm a *little* worse."

Just as he had predicted, he was never brought back to have his body offered up as evidence.

Females also underwent these medicalized exhibitions, but they do not write about them with the vividness male writers bring to them. Was it because they were more traumatized? In the 1950s physicians were almost universally male—was it so much more upsetting to have one's body displayed before the opposite sex? I think the reason men recall these scenes so vividly was the shock at having their bodies feminized, being turned from actors and doers into passive recipients of a male gaze.

A photograph in John Pohl's textbook about Sister Kenny's method speaks volumes: A girl on the verge of adolescence, her breasts just beginning to bud, wearing that garment that was a cross between a loincloth and a diaper, lies on a treatment table. Stately and plump and authoritative, Elizabeth Kenny is behind her, her gaze fixed on the girl's limb, which is being raised into the air. The girl, her head turned toward the camera, glares, rage and shame writ plainly on her face.

In the film *Sister Kenny,* disabled children are rendered as one-dimensional, negative object lessons. At one point Dr. McDonnell, Kenny's mentor, ushers Kenny down to a ward where children who have been left disabled as a result of the virus are playing. As he pauses at the door before opening it, background music starts to play, simultaneously warning and piteous. Then the door opens. From above we look down on a group of children. There is one, his body bent forward at the hips, his hands on the floor, pushing himself into an upright position. (It is the way I rise from the floor.) The camera pauses to stare: The child's frozen posture carries an inescapable suggestion of the simian. The mournful music that continues to play under the scene tells us that we are meant to experience this as a tragedy.

My eyes are experienced enough to know that these are not nondisabled child actors pretending to be disabled, but children disabled by polio. I wonder how they felt when they saw the film. I wonder if anyone gave a thought to how they would experience having their bodies displayed as objects of pity and terror. It is the first appearance of the figure of the crippled child in the film, and throughout the movie that passive figure will recur—a figure to be argued over, displayed, but generally kept mute. The one exception to that rule of utter passivity occurs shortly thereafter, when one child comes into Dr. Brack's office, filled with pride because he has learned how to kick a ball, and wants to show his new skill off to the doctor. In the terms of the film, we are meant to find David's pride poignant; yes, he can kick a ball—and can give it quite a kick too: he shatters the glass in one of Dr. Brack's display cabinets—but he's not like carefree Dory, with her dirty hands and dirty knees, romping about in her bloomers.

An exposé of charities—which ran, significantly, in *True: The Man's Magazine*—explicitly targeted the softheartedness of women as enabling crooked charities to exploit the community's goodwill:

> Your wife may have gotten one of these letters [soliciting a charitable contribution] during the day, while you were at work. She had the rest of the day to reflect on the touching appeal. After supper she might have gotten you your slippers and pipe, and, after you were both settled comfortably by the fire, she might have taken out the letter and showed it to you.
>
> "We're so lucky to be happy and well," she might have said gently. "Don't you think we could give $10 to help these blind people?"
>
> In your mellow mood, and because your wife wanted it, you might have taken out the checkbook, written the check, and handed it to her with a smile.
>
> If you didn't do this—then thousands of other husbands did.

Later in that same article women were again evoked—this time not as those who might seduce you into giving with tender words, pipes, and slippers, but as those marshaled by the National Foundation in their Mother's Marches, "female hordes" "whose function was to march into your living room and relieve you of as much money as they could get." In the 1950s, during the Korean War, the word "hordes" had taken on a specific association with the Chinese, whose army was often spoken of as "the Chinese hordes"—simultaneously Red and yellow.

Kenny had confronted a medical system that was overwhelmingly male, and quite determined to stay that way. Dr. John Pohl, the Minnesota orthopedist who later became one of Kenny's greatest supporters, had had his own experience of sexism. He'd first applied for medical school under the name he'd been given at birth—Florian Pohl, only to be rejected because it was assumed he was a woman. Only after changing his name to John Florian Pohl was he able to gain admittance to medical school.

It isn't only in the film *Sister Kenny* that we see polio playing havoc with expected gender roles. Charles Mee recalls arriving at the emergency room door when he first has polio and being wheeled into "This little band of panic" made up of nurses and orderlies. Mee was lifted onto a table, and "the crowd of nurses parted to let an immense red-haired woman, the head nurse, step forward, look at me lying on the table and pronounce without hesitation: 'This boy has polio.'" Mee—a fourteen-year-old 160-pound football player—found himself lifted up by this woman "strong as a linebacker for the Green Bay Packers" and borne "out of the examining room . . . into the immense quiet of the isolation ward."

Mee understood that this woman was risking getting polio herself. "A brave, heroic woman. I understood it the moment she picked me up. Mrs. Fuller was her name."

This was the 1950s, an era when heroism for women had gone the way of ration coupons and scrap-metal drives and blouses with shoulder pads. Here was a woman praised not only for her bravery but for her strength and heft and size. I'm struck by how often this image of female healer as Amazon or football player recurs in polio narratives. Edward Le Comte, a professor at Columbia who came down with polio on a sabbatical visit to France, describes his first physical therapist, Mme. Gautier:

. . . . an inspiring sight to the bedridden, for she was a large, bouncy, equine woman. . . . She kept up a tireless flow of imperfect English . . . hoisted me with one Amazonian arm. . . . The next part of the hour was given to massage. This Mme. Gautier performed in great sweeping waves.

And Sister Kenny, you'll recall, was described as looking "like a good blocking back at Notre Dame."

SURVIVAL SKILLS

My parents had sometimes threatened to send Sandra to Northfield, a boarding school where an old friend from our Hamilton days was headmaster, hoping this would save her from hanging around with boys my father referred to as "drugstore cowboys." When I was thirteen I said that I wanted to go to Northfield.

"What the fuck do you want to go there for?" Sandra said.

I normally wouldn't disagree with Sandra about anything. If she hated a popular song, I hated it, too. If she declared that girls who wore V-neck sweaters without a blouse underneath looked cheap, then I thought just the same about the scandalous amount of flesh shown by such girls. I wore my hair just like Sandra's—long and straight, parted far on the left side, so that a hank of it drooped across our right eyes. Grownups would say that we looked like Veronica Lake, a forties film actress who had worn her hair in a similar fashion.

That I was willing to risk Sandra's scorn spoke of how desperate I was to flee that house.

All through junior high school I'd been hearing from my classmates about the near-miraculous properties of diet pills, as Dexedrine, a type of amphetamine, was known. The summer before I started at Northfield, I got my mother to take me to my pediatrician, a man with enormous bushy eyebrows and a lantern jaw who bore more than a passing resemblance to

Herman Munster. Although he said I didn't look as if I needed to go on a diet, and that my weight was within normal limits, he was willing to prescribe them for me. The ease with which he dashed off this prescription wasn't unusual then. Pep pills—Dexedrine was known as one—were also handed out to counter any number of ailments, including "pregnancy blahs."

After filling the prescription for the diet pills, my mother said, "Oh, it's the vertical stripes on that dress you're wearing. That's why he thought you didn't need to lose weight." Looking back I once again find myself in a situation where it is nearly impossible for me to parse the reactions within my family. When my mother was so sure that I needed to lose weight, despite what the weight chart said, was that because she had grown used to thinking of my body as something that needed to be changed, fixed, healed? Or was it because of the general fear of female flesh that seemed to ooze out of my father's pores, circulating through our home like a toxic gas—so that it would just be better if there were less of it, of me? How do I tease apart the culture's general disdain for disabled bodies and the effects of rehab that had convinced me that my body was a foreign land to be subjugated to my will?

I swallowed the first of the diet pills the next morning. The idea of breakfast seemed repulsive, and at lunch, I was full after a few bites of grilled Velveeta on white bread. I barely picked at dinner. When I stepped on the scale the next morning, I had lost three pounds. The miraculousness of these pills wasn't just in the way weight seemed to stream off my body: The depression that had been shadowing me for the last patch of my life lifted, as suddenly and decisively as a theater curtain being rung up. I slept four or five hours a night—but who needed sleep? It was a waste of time. Suddenly everything seemed possible: I would become one of the New York City career girls I'd read about in *Glamour* and *Cosmopolitan*. That child, struggling for breath as the ether mask came down over her face, struggling for breath as her father's hands pressed down against her windpipe, bore no relation to the cool and confident young woman I was bound to become. In the speed-fueled fantasies I was striding down Fifth Avenue in New York City, miraculously crutchless, not limping, in a perfectly matched outfit, on my way from my office—I worked in film or advertising—to my apartment (the word "apartment" seemed the most exciting word in the English language), where my boyfriend, a man named Scott or Mitchell, would shortly arrive. Scott or

Mitchell would have hazel eyes, a square jaw, and two dozen long-stemmed red roses for me. Dexedrine was a can-do, all-American drug, one that not only promised quick and easy transformation but seemed to deliver it.

I didn't realize how much of my mood was a result of the medication. I seemed to be spiraling upward, my weight loss making me more confident, my confidence making me want to strive harder to become the perfect person I was meant to be.

As the summer drew to a close, my weight plateaued, about five pounds above what I had decided was my ideal weight, and nothing I did could get the needle on the scale to move in the slightest to the left. That wonderful world in which I would be thin and glamorous and perfect hovered just beyond my reach.

The first night at boarding school the lights went out promptly at nine o'clock, and, as darkness descended on the freshman dorm, the sounds of homesick girls sobbing drifted down the hallways. The crying seemed to be contagious. My roommate, Mary, soon joined in, muffling her sobs in her pillow. How could girls so old be homesick? I had felt a strange sort of pity for them, my pity shadowed with contempt. I was so far beyond all that. Giving a world-weary shrug of my shoulders, I turned on my side and stared out the window. I did not allow myself to know the envy I felt for those who longed for their absent families, those for whom this was the first taste of homesickness. The bells in the campus chapel rang out not just the hour, but the quarter hours, too. I heard ten and eleven strike, and the quarter hours in between; and then midnight and one, too, before I finally fell asleep.

After a week of lying awake for hours and hours after lights out, I decided to stop taking the diet pills, especially since they no longer seemed to be doing anything for my weight. While I never slept for the ten hours Northfield expected us to, I no longer lay awake for half the night.

My body, released from its chemically induced bout of starvation, behaved as evolution had taught it, fattening itself up against the possibility of lean times to come. The food served at boarding school was lush compared to what I was used to at home. My mother's approach to cooking had always been only slightly to the left of utilitarian. A few years before, my aunt Dorothy—my mother's good sister, the one who never had dust bunnies under her sofa and who served homemade English muffins for breakfast and sent out thousands of Christmas cards—had given my mother a cookbook called *The I Hate to Cook Book*. Part storehouse of quick and easy recipes, part protest against the mystique of the happy housewife, the book had recipes for dishes like "Skid Row Stroganoff" and "Stayabed Stew." My mother adored the book and added quotes from it to her repertoire: "When in doubt, throw it out," and "I'll bring the water for the lemonade."

Most of the recipes she cooked from it were mixtures of hamburger, frozen vegetables, and canned soups, either mushroom or tomato, which simmered in the oven all day and filled me with a sense of despair when I came home from school in the afternoon and found their odors wafting through the house. Accompanying Stayabed Stew might be a salad of iceberg lettuce, dressed with a salad dressing made from Good Seasons packaged mix to which corn oil and the store brand of apple cider vinegar had been added.

When my father was in a good mood, he'd joke at the end of the meal, "What's for dessert tonight, Mary El? Baked Alaska?" We rarely had dessert, and certainly never baked Alaska—ice cream covered with meringue and popped in a very hot oven—that had been the specialty at a resort in Maine where my father had worked as a waiter during the summers when he was a teenager. If, at the end of a meal, we said we were still hungry, my mother would tell us to have a piece of fruit, although the fruit she bought was prepackaged in plastic bags, baking apples and oranges designed for juicing.

At Northfield we not only had dessert with both lunch and dinner but coffee cake for breakfast some mornings, and mashed potatoes—real potatoes, not instant—formed into peaks and glazed with grated cheese, or served in a mound, with a pool of butter, not margarine, melting in a caldera on top. The weight that had poured away from my frame now poured back. The seams of my blouses bound against my armpits; buttons popped off.

Of course no one had warned me that stopping the diet pills would result in a plummet from my months-long high. Just as I hadn't attributed my elevated mood to the diet pills, so I wasn't able to make the connection that the crash that followed was caused by withdrawal. My post-Dexedrine depression was exacerbated by the fact that the academic standards at an exclusive prep school were far more rigorous than what I was used to. When I turned in my first tests and papers—work that would have earned me an A at Nathan Bishop Junior High—the papers were returned to me with bright red Fs and Ds scrawled on them.

Northfield—originally known as the Northfield Seminary for Young Ladies—had been founded in the late nineteenth century by evangelist Dwight L. Moody to educate the genteel poor of all races. His Victorian legacy survived, not only in the physical appearance of the campus— several of the buildings, dating from the school's founding, were of red brick, with turrets, sharply slanted roofs, and gingerbread trim beneath the eaves—but also in the school's overall ambiance and customs. Our lives were hemmed in by an enormous number of rules—for instance, while one might wear pants on Saturdays, it was forbidden to walk past the nearby Northfield Inn while wearing them. Pants could not—of course!—be worn on Sundays, nor could laundry be done on that day. This was one of the many rules I inadvertently violated, only to be met with the housemother saying to me, in a shocked tone of voice, "Your mother wouldn't do wash on Sundays, would she?" The school honor code might have been written by Joseph Stalin in collaboration with Joseph McCarthy. Not only was a student who violated any of the school rules required to turn herself in and confess her misdeeds, but anyone who was aware of a violation by another and failed to report the errant behavior was deemed equally guilty.

In addition to keeping the Sabbath and comporting ourselves in a ladylike manner, we were also expected to perform daily chores. These daily duties—I was assigned to washing the dishes after dinner—were known as "dummy," and the shapeless coveralls we wore while performing our daily physical labor were called "dummy smocks." If we complained about dummy, one of the senior girls who lived in the freshman dorm and watched over us was sure to tell us about the days when Northfield girls had had to rise at dawn to milk the school's herd of cows.

Hand in hand with this clean-scrubbed ardor and sense of rectitude was a commitment on the part of many of the students and staff to social justice. Miss Howland, a religion teacher who lived in my dorm, went most weekends to New Haven, where she was involved, along with others from the religious left, in antiwar and community organizing projects. The neighborhoods she moved around in New Haven were tough enough that at night she walked around with a doorknob in a sock, which could be used to kibosh muggers. She dressed with a sort of defiant frumpiness, wearing one of a collection of jumpers—bibbed skirts worn with a blouse underneath—in red, black, or navy; sometimes wearing the same outfit for three or even four days running; and her hair was shorn Prince Valiant style, with straight bangs. Despite Miss Howland's dowdiness, she was idolized by the girls who were rebels.

The school divided itself into three rough social groupings: the already-jaded future debutantes, who could talk at length about different brands of skis and tennis racquets and their opinions of various beaches in the Caribbean; the good girls, who might tear up when the our school song was sung in chapel ("O Northfield beautiful! O Northfield dear and fair! Loyal and dutiful, thy daughters everywhere."); and then the rebels, who dressed in blue jean jackets and skirts, who loved Thomas Pynchon and hated LBJ and his war.

I aligned myself with the wearers of blue jean jackets and blue jean skirts, although I owned neither of those items. I went to meetings of the social action club, which held car washes to raise money to send to civil rights workers in the South. I idolized one of its senior members, who befriended me. She lived in New York, and sometimes went to a bookstore where a magazine called *Fuck You: A Magazine of the Arts* was published. It was even rumored that she had actually had sex. I had nothing but contempt for the self I had planned on becoming six months previously—the woman with the manicured nails and perfectly cut hair striding along Fifth Avenue between her glamorous job in advertising and her fashionable apartment. My fantasies still involved New York, but now they involved cluttered art-filled flats on the Lower East Side and conversations about truth and justice that would stretch long into the night, as my friends and I smoked too many cigarettes and drank too much cheap red wine. I said that Thomas Pynchon was my favorite writer, although the truth was I hadn't been able to get beyond the first page of *V*.

Opposition to the Vietnam War was intermingled with patrician disdain for Lyndon Baines Johnson, a graduate not of Columbia or Harvard but of Southwest Texas State Teachers College; LBJ with his Texas drawl and his coarse country habits—picking up his beagle by its floppy ears, lifting up his shirt in front of photographers to show off the incision from recent gallbladder surgery.

Since it took me roughly three times as long to get between classes as it took my fellow students, I almost invariably arrived in class late, out of breath, and even in the dead of winter, sweating. The ice and snow of a New England winter didn't make things any easier, but I was used to going through the winter with a good collection of bruises from slipping on ice. Sometimes the pathways shoveled through the snow were so narrow that the only way I could maneuver along them was by swinging my crutches up over my head in enormous circles. Climbing stairs had never been any more difficult for me than walking—it was just another activity that I accomplished a lot more slowly and with a lot more effort than everyone else around me.

I had carefully tidied my dorm room for the first of the weekly inspections that would be carried out by our housemother—a most unmaternal woman named Winifred Trask. I looked around my half of the shared room, proud of how perfectly neat I had managed to make it. My mother would have been delighted if my room at home had ever been in such an uncluttered state. But when I returned at lunch, there would be the written result of Miss Trask's inspection on my desk, a list of my failings with a red D at the top. My wastebasket had not been emptied, my bedspread was wrinkled, and my shoes were jumbled on the floor of the closet. It hadn't occurred to me that I should have set them so that the soles rested on the floor, in matching pairs, with the left shoe on the left side and the right shoe on the right, or that a bed should not just be made but made flawlessly. I thought I had learned my lesson, but the scenario kept repeating itself. I'd look around the room every Friday morning, certain that *this* time I'd figured it out, and unable to see a single thing that Miss Trask might fault me on. But every Friday I'd return to Weston Hall for lunch and find that list of ways in which I had once again failed to rise to Miss Trask's standards.

Once my roommate, Mary, exasperated at the state of our room, said to me, "You know, there are two other girls at this school who have the same problem you do." I felt flooded with relief. It wasn't just me; I wasn't the only one whose dorm room looked impeccable to her and slovenly to the housemother.

And then Mary said, "Just because you're . . ." When Mary paused, the way people always did before they said the word "handicapped" or "had polio," the relief I had felt vanished. As always, any problem I had always and inevitably became *that* problem.

In eighth grade our class had been allowed to organize a dance at Nathan Bishop, and I had planned to go with Tommy Johnson, who lived down the street from me and went to Holy Name. I knew the other girls would find Tommy so cute that they'd be envious of me. He was an Irish Huck Finn, with freckles across his nose and long, beautiful eyelashes. I practiced dancing in front of the full-length mirror in my room, imitating the swinging of arms and swaying of hips I'd seen Sandra do, although I kept my feet firmly planted on the floor—if I tried to move them as I gyrated the upper two-thirds of my body to "Please Mr. Postman" or "Stop! In the Name of Love," I'd stumble. Would people think I was strange if I danced? Or would they think I was strange if I didn't dance? As Saturday drew closer I grew more and more anxious. The enormous good fortune of Tommy having consented to go with me made me feel jittery, too. I knew that when I entered the gym with him an immediate female chorus of whispers would start: "He's *cute*." "He came with *Anne*." On the evening of the dance I said I had a terrible headache and stayed home.

At the beginning of the semester, mixers were held between the freshman girls of Northfield and the freshman boys of Mount Hermon. I went and stood, leaning on my crutches, with the rest of the wallflowers. At home, at least, boys had gotten to know me by sitting next to me in class and hanging out with me in groups after class. I try to imagine what kind of fourteen-year-old boy would have risked his schoolmates' scorn and his own discomfort to walk across that room and ask me to dance.

When I went home for a weekend visit, Sandra said to me: "If we see a penny lying on the ground, we pick it up because this family is so poor—because you are going to boarding school." She said "boarding school" with the same snarl of contempt with which many of my new classmates said the word "public school." To this day I will bend over—no matter how much pain it causes me, how difficult it is—and pick up any coins I see lying on the sidewalk. I was in my thirties before I could go grocery shopping without feeling battered by waves of remorse as I pushed my

shopping cart through the doors of Safeway toward my car, silently repri-
manding myself for not living frugally on a diet of cabbage and tofu.

I was too guilt ridden to ask my parents for any money. I even started
skimping on doing my laundry, afraid to spend quarters on the washing
machines and dryers in the basement of Weston Hall. Of course walking
was such an effort that I worked up a good sweat just making my way
from one classroom building to another and then back to my dorm, so
that my clothes soon began to reek of my dank body odor. When one of
the seniors who lived in the freshmen dorms told me that I smelled
("Sometimes when you come in the room it almost bowls me over"), I
sobbed with shame. I couldn't stop sobbing for days.

I called my parents from the phone booth outside the dorm. "I can't
stop crying," I managed to say. My mother was her usual chipper self,
reeling off some of the handy catchphrases she used on such occasions.
Did she tell me, "Into each life some rain must fall," or "Life isn't a bowl
of cherries," or "Don't make a mountain out of a molehill"?

"Let me talk to Daddy."

I knew I might catch him in a mood where he'd tell me, "You've made
your poor mother cry" in a pathetic voice or "You just ruin everything,
don't you?" But I also knew I might luck out and find him in a state where
he'd respond to me.

"What's wrong, sweetie?" It was early in the evening, after a few martinis had smoothed away the edge of anger that built up in him each day
and before alcohol's lubrication had made him so loose that each word he
spoke took twice as long as usual to utter.

"I don't know." I tucked the black receiver between my shoulder and
the side of my head, and wiped my nose and eyes with the scratchy woolen
sleeve of my duffel coat. After a few minutes, I said, "Everything."

I kept crying. My father said, "Maybe you need to see a psychiatrist."

My visual images of psychiatry had been formed from *New Yorker*
cartoons. When my father said those words, I imagined myself lying on a
couch, with a goateed doctor off to one side, holding a pad and pencil,
and an inevitable potted palm in the background. I pictured a sage and in-
finitely understanding man who would be able to instantly cure whatever
was so disastrously wrong in my life.

"Do you want us to come up and see you?"

"Yes," I said. I could scarcely believe his concern, his willingness to
take me seriously. Later on, I realized that my father can be empathic and

deeply generous when another person's suffering matches his own. Once, when I was in my mid-forties, he asked me how my health was. I was surprised he'd asked me the question, and began to tell him—gently, carefully, so as not to alarm him—about the increasing fatigue I was experiencing from postpolio syndrome. He cut me off: "I meant your asthma," he said, referring to our shared bane.

And once my father called me, telling me he was going to buy me a stair lift I needed but hadn't been able to afford. "My hip's been hurting me, walking up the stairs," he said. "I want to buy you a stair lift."

When I called from that phone booth at Northfield, he must have heard some echo of himself, lost and floundering. But as so often happened in our family, that conversation was swallowed up in the vast sea of silence in which we lived. The promised visit never materialized, and nothing was done about getting me help. Perhaps my mother had said, in her way that was half dismissive, half pacifying, "Oh, Jack, she'll be all right. She's just being a teenager." Or perhaps the wash of predinner martinis, the after-dinner highball, endlessly freshened throughout the evening, had rubbed away the rough edges of that conversation so that, when they recalled it the next morning, what had been said was only vaguely remembered.

My mother continued to send me newsy letters—reporting on the weather and my sisters' and brother's school activities—that seemed to come from a family that existed only in her imagination.

Home for spring break, I picked up a flyer about an upcoming antiwar demonstration from a stack in the parish house of the First Unitarian Church. I read every word of the flyer, mimeographed onto bright yellow paper, and then folded it in quarters and stashed it in the pocket of my brown duffel coat, resolving to go to the demonstration, which would be held in about a week. Throughout the week I would thrust my hand into the pocket and touch the flyer, repeating my promise to myself to go, all the time half afraid that I might end up by allowing my fear to overtake me at the last minute, as it had the day of the eighth-grade dance.

Walking in that scraggly picket line seemed the most exciting thing I had ever done. And then one of the demonstrators, a Pembroke or RISD student, with wild and curly long hair and gold hoop earrings, moved up and down the picket line, saying to various friends of hers: "Party—my apartment." "I'm having a party. After the demonstration."

I tried to imagine the party, the apartment itself. Would there be a poster of Che Guevara on the wall? Candles burning? How I longed to go to such a party, to be a real part of that world!

I didn't go back to Northfield after my freshman year. Partly it was my guilt about the amount of money it was costing my parents, but mostly it was out of my desire to take part in the antiwar movement. My father's violence seemed to have abated. He never got on top of me and choked me again, although I have a vague memory of his kicking me down the stairs. Did that really happen? It is one of those memories so fragmentary that I wonder if it's true. And I always think of that incident that Jane remembers, of my father throwing me out of the room and pulling my mother in, while she yelled, "Run! Get out of the house!"—an incident which I have completely blocked from my memory. I do know that throughout my adult life, when a visit from my parents has been imminent, I have a repeated image of myself being kicked down a flight of stairs.

MARCHING ON THE PENTAGON

I suppose I didn't march on the Pentagon, if we accept the dictionary's definition of the word "march": "to move along steadily, usually with a rhythmic stride and in step with others." First off, there was my lack of steadiness, the fact that I needed, as I made my way along the route between the Lincoln Memorial and the Pentagon, to drop to the sidelines for a few minutes and rest, recovering from my exhaustion. And certainly my mode of ambulation—*Life* magazine would later describe it as exhibiting "excruciating coordination"—could hardly be described as striding. I planted my crutches ahead of me, and, lifting up both my feet, swung my whole body forward. It wasn't the way physical therapists liked me to walk—they always told me to move one crutch and one foot at a time, so that my gait would more closely approximate normal walking—but while my way of walking was slow, theirs was far slower and much more tiring. And as for my rhythm? No John Philip Souza tempo; the music for my version of marching might have been played by John Cage or John Coltrane, with its own strange syncopation.

At fifteen "almost sixteen," as I said in those days, in 1967, I started my junior year of high school. I wore a new-for-the-first-day-of-school dress that had bold stripes of orange and brick red and yellow. I also wore a black-and-white button pinned to my chest that said "Confront the War-makers—October 21—March on the Pentagon," wearing it above my left breast—where, a few years before, my oldest sister had worn a circle pin made of ersatz gold.

But wait. I do remember that first-day-of-school dress, with its bold stripes: Girls had to wear skirts or dresses to school, and everyone had a new one to start the year, whether it was bought at the upscale shop Poise'N'Ivy in Barrington or via layaway, a dollar down and a dollar a week, at Zayre's or Lerner's. The more I think about it, I'm not so sure I wore that dress the first day of my junior year in high school. Maybe it was my sophomore year?

I expected that when I got to this point in my life, my memories would unroll in a smooth, glitchless narrative. But it's not a well-plotted movie that reels at a regular speed through the projector. Instead it's like looking at jumbled snapshots, pulled randomly out of the box where they had been stored. The images themselves are clear—here I am, unwrapping the aluminum foil from around the tuna fish sandwich that was meant to be my lunch on the charter bus on the way to a demonstration. But was that on the day we went to Washington to march on the Pentagon? Or was it earlier, in April of that same year? Were the buses heading not to Washington but to an antiwar demonstration in New York?

Several times I'd gotten up at four thirty or five in the morning—my mother, having been the one to set her alarm, would open my bedroom door and say, "Anne, time to get up." On school mornings she had to prod me over and over again to get me out of bed, but I'd arise immediately on these days. As I came down the stairs, I must have heard the *slurp-plunk, slurp-plunk* of the coffee percolator; maybe even, since the house so early in the morning would have been unusually still, the sound of my mother's worn slippers on the linoleum floor as she moved about the kitchen, unloading dishes from the dishwasher or pouring me orange juice. She would have been wearing her cotton pajamas and ancient bathrobe. My mother is of the generation that keeps things: She still has the steam iron she used all through our childhood, its frayed cord repaired with duct tape by my father—a slipshod but serviceable job; the towels hanging in my parents' bathroom must be several decades old.

When she dropped me at the corner in downtown Providence where the charter buses were lined up and waiting for us, I don't remember if she said, "Be careful," or "I'm proud of you." I don't think she said either. She had retreated into a world of stubborn silence. Sometimes weeks went by when the only words she said directly to me were, "Pick up your coat." Partly I dropped my coat on the floor every day when I came home from school because I was exhausted by the walk home, but partly I dropped my coat on the floor so she would at least say to me, "Anne Finger, how many times do I have to tell you—pick up your coat!"

Knots of people were waiting on that corner in the peculiar thin light of early morning as it leeched from late, late night. The buses' engines were running but their doors were not yet opened. The waiting male demonstrators wore neckties and jackets; the women, dresses. We did not want to alienate people by failing to look respectable. A few demonstrators balanced the clutch of hand-drawn signs we had turned out at a sign-making party a few nights before. Hands were rubbed together against the cold; breath was visible in the air. Maybe the drivers didn't open the bus doors because they were disdainful of antiwar protesters and didn't want to make things any easier for us. Or maybe they didn't want their workday to start any earlier than it had to—didn't want to have to start answering our questions: *When will we be leaving? How long is it going to take us to get there? When will we have a rest stop?* When they saw me on my crutches, though, one of them might have gestured to me and let me on the bus, the doors giving off a slight wheeze as they opened. "Just her," they might have said, although if Faith was with me, I'd have said, "She's my friend," and they'd have let her on, too.

It had all started to seem ritualized—gathering in the half-light of early dawn; being lulled by the rhythm of the road and drifting back to sleep around Kingston or Westerly; the march itself; the speeches. We protested; the war escalated. We protested again; the war escalated again.

The March on the Pentagon was going to be different. We were going to go to the heart of the beast, not to some safe and distant area where we would hear speakers saying the expected things and then go home. We were going to confront the war makers. Anything might happen. There were rumors that troops—not just policemen with batons at the ready, riot helmets, and holstered guns, not just the weekend warriors of the National Guard, but regular U.S. Army troops, with rifles and bayonets—would be there to protect the Pentagon.

That August and September and October, when my weekly *National Guardian* arrived—a rather strange title for a leftist newspaper, which it nonetheless was—I would take it up to my bedroom and read it eagerly. The newspaper had been founded in 1948, in the midst of the post–World War II anti-Communist hysteria—which preceded and outlasted the phenomenon known as McCarthyism. Founded by people who were sympathetic to the Communist Party but not directly aligned with it, the news weekly had no doubt hoped to invoke by its name the Popular Front period of the 1930s, when opposition to fascism had been the overwhelming concern, and divisions between leftists and liberals had been played down. In 1948 the name *National Guardian* had meant to suggest that the paper was guarding the national ideals of Jefferson and Lincoln. But by the mid-1960s, with the National Guard being called onto college campuses and into cities to put down uprisings in the black community, the name didn't just seem fuddy-duddy, it seemed positively bizarre. In the September 9, 1967, issue, one of the articles was headlined "SNCC Leader Asks for Guns." SNCC—pronounced "Snick"—stood for "Student Nonviolent Coordinating Committee," a group that had played a key role in the bloody freedom rides to integrate Greyhound and other bus lines in the south.

In the summer of 1965 I'd staffed an antiwar booth that had collected money and proselytized at the Newport Jazz Festival. The booth next to us was doing the same thing for SNCC. Our booth, in those early days of the antiwar movement, was staffed mostly by Quakers in sensible shoes. The women had solid, motherly hips and wore flowing dresses, and the men had wispy untrimmed beards. I looked over with envy at the organizers from SNCC, both black and white, who were known as "SNCC kids." Some of them spoke with the drawls of the Deep South. They were all lithe and wore jeans and tight-fitting denim jackets. To be a civil rights organizer in the South meant to live a heroic life, filled with ever-present risk. The summer before, when three civil rights workers were murdered in Mississippi, the hunt for their bodies turned up more than a dozen other dumped bodies—black men bound with wire and rope, tossed into rivers, leaving behind survivors too terrified to report their deaths. I wanted to live the way the SNCC kids lived, in crowded ramshackle houses in Mississippi or Georgia or Alabama, I wanted to be brave— really brave, not just called brave for going about my life. I wanted to sleep on a lumpy mattress on the floor. I wanted to serve myself a plate of rice and black-eyed peas from a simmering pot on the stove. I knew that I couldn't have those things at the age of fifteen—I supposed that when I was eighteen I'd be old enough to head for the South and be an organizer. Three years seemed to be forever.

One thing I could have was a tight-fitting blue denim jacket like the ones they wore. How did I find out that they sold such jackets at Sears Roebuck? I must have dared to ask someone—surely not one of the SNCC kids themselves, to whom I spoke only with great reluctance out of fear that I would embarrass myself by saying something stupid. I finally got my mother to take me to the Sears Roebuck store on North Main Street. Stores weren't open in the evening then. With relatively few women in the paid workforce, it was assumed that shopping could be done between the hours of ten and five thirty. My mother was always promising to take me places in the afternoon but ended up canceling over and over and over again—a meeting at school or having to cover a class for a colleague. Finally, after weeks of postponed plans, she took me to Sears. I looked all through the section where they displayed work clothes—painters' pants and coveralls, stiff-legged denim blue jeans. I found a jacket that was something like the ones the SNCC kids had worn, but not exactly—it was a lighter blue, and baggier. I went back and forth. No, it wasn't quite right; I shouldn't buy it. I should buy it—I'd regret it later, and it would be so hard to get my mother to bring me back here. Finally I did get it, but when I got home and stood in front of the full-length mirror in my bedroom, I felt nothing but sadness. I didn't look like the SNCC kids, I just looked like me.

Under that headline, "SNCC Leader Asks for Guns," H. Rap Brown warned demonstrators at the Pentagon "to expect the worst from the police. 'If you believe the police aren't going to come down like the Gestapo, you're deluding yourselves.'"

That summer there had been riots—on the left we were beginning to call them uprisings and rebellions—in cities all across the country, the largest in Detroit and Newark. In Detroit, the National Guard had been unable to bring the city under control, and the Eighty-second Airborne had been called in. In Newark, ten million dollars' worth of property was destroyed in four days. Columns of smoke rose from cities; the sound of rifle fire was heard. The days when we had gathered singing, "We Shall Overcome," crossing our arms one over the other and taking the hand of the person next to us and, swaying back and forth en masse singing, "Black and white together . . ." seemed to belong to ancient history.

The *Guardian* posed the question: "What should white radicals do in response to ghetto rebellions?" ending with the response from author John Gerassi, "My answer is, support them, and I mean militarily." The *National Guardian* also ran a full-page ad for a new magazine to be called *Avant-Garde*. Beneath a picture of a long-haired, barefoot woman in an op art dress, with her arms stretched over her head and a sex-kittenish pout on her face, were the words A PROPOSITION. For many years I had been under the impression that the term "avant-garde" was pronounced "ah-VANT gar-DEZ"—which shows how much—or, more accurately, how little—attention I paid in French class. Fortunately I had said the word aloud in front of my mother and sister Susan, who had let me know of my gaffe—far better to have them laughing at me than anyone else.

"A wild new thing is about to happen," the copy read. "As its name implies, *Avant-Garde* will be a forward-directed, daring, and wildly hedonistic magazine." The table of contents for the premiere issue listed articles such as, "Understanding Zowie—A Glossary of Switched-On Generation Jargon," "The Prison Poems of Ho Chi Minh," and Julian Huxley's "A Plea for State-Sponsored Breeding of Supermen."

I imagined a world in which, during a lull in gunfire at the barricades, I might pull a book of poems by Ho Chi Minh from my jacket pocket—not the pale blue denim jacket I had bought at Sears but the exact jacket the SNCC kids wore.

Later my friend Suzanne, who went to RISD and whom I idolized as I had once idolized my sister Sandra, looked at that same ad and snorted, and I was instantly ashamed of myself for ever having thought it seemed cool. To the world outside I looked so brave and bold, but inside I felt so lost, so eager to be the coolest, the most revolutionary, and so certain that I was not.

I was so often lost in the intellectual wilderness of the New Left. Unlike the Old Left, where there had been the dominant catechism of the Communist Party and then the dissenting ideologies of the groups op-posed to the Communist Party, the New Left was a free-for-all, and I sometimes felt as if I were drowning in that morass. There was no easy rope for me to hold on to. I had tried to read Marx, but I found myself lost. I thought that perhaps I needed to be grounded in Hegelianism, the philosophy Marx had used as his jumping-off point. I used someone's library card to take Hegel's *Phenomenology* from the Brown Library, but got through just the first couple of sentences. I am only glad that no one told me that in order to understand Hegel one had to read him in the original German—because then I would no doubt have gotten a beginning German textbook and set out to teach myself the language, diligently folding a piece of blue-lined notebook paper in half and writing German vocabulary words on the left side of the fold and their English translations on the right, copying out irregular conjugations. I would have been gung-ho for a day or two, putting in three or four hours a night—and hiding what I was doing from the rest of my family so I wouldn't get teased. Soon I would have been distracted by other things, and the neatly written lists of German vocabulary words, the handwritten conjugations, the nouns I had practiced declining would all have been buried under piles of other pieces of paper on my desk—homework assignments I had begun and abandoned, or which I had finished and forgotten to bring to school, copies of the *Guardian*, half-read paperback books—perhaps of Hermann Hesse's *Demian* or Frantz Fanon's *The Wretched of the Earth.*

My parents had been concerned enough about the militancy of the March on the Pentagon that they had at first forbidden me to go. Our discussions would have begun with me promising to be careful and not to get arrested—and ended with my making an analogy between Lyndon Baines Johnson and Adolf Hitler (no political discussion could happen without it), and the *extremis* of the current moment with that of a generation before, when complacent Europeans had failed to stop fascism. In this familial psychohistorical drama my parents, of course, played the role of the staid and comfortable bourgeoisie who had deluded themselves into thinking that Hitler was a flash-in-the-pan, a buffoon. I, of course, was the passionate-but-nonetheless-clear-eyed young radical. Of course in the novels I'd read and the movies I'd seen, these dedicated and insightful radicals were always male. The women were invariably attached to a man, and their loyalty to the cause was channeled through him. I could imagine a man in one of these narratives who walked with a stiff-legged limp and leaned on a cane as a result of a war wound. It was completely impossible to imagine a female walking in such a way unless she was a good-hearted dowager, playing a role peripheral to the action, perhaps hiding the dashing young Resistance hero and his dewy-eyed companion in her cellar or in the hayloft of her barn.

While I argued with my parents about whether or not I was going to the demonstration, I continued organizing for it, arranging for the charter buses, attending endless meetings, getting out the word—which mostly consisted of producing flyers to be passed out and copying them on a recalcitrant mimeograph machine, which always left splotches of black ink on my hands, and on my face as I pushed my long hair back from it with my ink-stained fingers.

A few months before the October march, Abbie Hoffman and some of the other Yippies had joined a tour of the New York Stock Exchange. As was appropriate for a Yippie action, what happened next passed almost immediately into myth, and the facts became impossible to ascertain: One account had it that they had flung money down onto the trading floor, causing the traders below to leap into the air and lunge at one another as they grabbed for the dollar bills raining down on them. In another version Abbie had showed his contempt for money by setting a bill—variously rumored to be a hundred-dollar bill, a twenty-dollar bill, a five-dollar bill— on fire.

No matter what had happened, I disapproved of the Yippies' action. That money could have been given to the movement; it could have been put to good use. In truth I was both drawn to and frightened by the antics of the Yippies. I thought I had thrown off all the dead hands of the past, but I still had within me my parents' dour Yankee suspicious attitude toward money. On the one hand one ought to have enough of it, for being broke suggested that one was lazy and imprudent, but on the other using the words "money" and "fun" in the same sentence was unthinkable.

Abbie Hoffman, Allen Ginsberg, and the other Yippies had recently declared that they intended to surround the Pentagon, chant, and levitate it three hundred feet into the air. They had actually applied for a permit to do this and been granted one by that rare species, a bureaucrat with a sense of humor: The permit had been issued with the proviso that the Pentagon be lifted no more than ten feet in the air. Their proposed action was a jocular foray aimed at the war makers, but it was also directed at the increasingly militant and stern ethos of the Left.

I had finally persuaded my parents to allow me to go to the march. There was a proviso that I was to stay well back from the front lines and be under the protective care of one of my mother's friends, who was also going.

On that October morning my mother opened my bedroom door and said, "Anne, time to get up." Once again I drank a cup of Maxwell House coffee poured from the electric percolator and waited on a cold street corner in the early morning light to board a charter bus. On the bus two women in the seat behind me were discussing the possibility of getting in a trip to the National Gallery while they were in Washington. I was horrified. Napalm was raining down on the heads of the peasants of Vietnam, and they were talking about going to a *museum*!

I imagine that somewhere on I-95, perhaps near the exit for Wakefield or the one for Westerly, I fell back asleep. When I woke up on the bus between Providence and Washington somewhere near New Haven, maybe, did I slip straight from the world of dreaming into the world of daydreams? I imagine I did. Although I have no memories of using my daydreams as a way to escape from the boredom of lying in bed in the hospital, I have no doubt that it was there that my private theater began. Throughout most of my high school years, while I was lying in bed waiting for sleep to overtake me, or in classes that bored me, like geometry and French, on car trips, I would spin out fantasies that made Walter Mitty's daydreams seem tame. I was a savior of whole nations, a key actor in the liberation of the human race.

Sometimes I would be in a South American country where I had played a decisive role in overthrowing a brutal dictatorship. The oppressed people—who had lived for generations in poverty and hunger and fear—thronged into the streets. Their lifetimes lived in misery and want had burnished them free of all that was petty and ignoble. The faces in the crowd appeared to me frozen, like faces on a poster or in a still from movies about revolutionary struggle like *The Battle of Algiers* or *La Guerre Est Finie.*

My fantasies were rich with the imagined romance of being a revolutionary: the secret meetings, the brutal realities of power, the omnipresent possibility of death, the raw adrenaline of risk; even the comfort one could find in a world in which right and wrong were so sharply delineated. I ruminated on set pieces and played them over again and again as my Catholic schoolmates did the stations of the cross. There was the moment at the border where one was stopped, the clandestine passing of papers on a crowded trolley car, the prison, and of course the triumphant finale: the victorious masses thronging the streets. With all these wild fantasies going on, no wonder I rarely had any idea of what the geometry teacher was talking about and thought that the "avant-garde" was pronounced "ah-VANT Gar-DEZ"!

Sometimes in my fantasies I would be caught and tortured. The torture would be carried out in a basement, of course—I had watched enough movies to know that it was impossible for torture to be carried out anywhere except underground. The exact means of torture would be vague—electricity to my genitals, being hung upside down by my feet, having my head held underwater until I was at the point of drowning—and my own bodily sensations even more so. Yet certain things in that cellarlike space were in sharp focus: the green-shaded bulb, hanging from a wire in the center of the ceiling and casting a cone of light; the battered metal desk behind which the *jefe* would sit; the steepling of his fingers. Needless to say under this despicable torture I would be brave—unbelievably brave. The foreign revolutionaries, who generally held us *norteamericanos* in contempt, would make an exception for me, finding me worthy not just of their acceptance but of their admiration.

Perhaps I was yearning for the safely Manichaean world, a world in which good and evil were cleanly demarcated, that seemed to have existed shortly before my birth: that world in which a public address system had broadcast across Harvard Yard, as faithfully as a muezzin crying out the hour of prayer: "The uniform of the day will be the regular uniform of the day"; a world in which my mother's oft-repeated line from *Henry V*—"We few, we happy few, we band of brothers"—might echo without irony in the heads of soldiers trapped behind enemy lines.

Did I walk on crutches in those fantasies? I think I conveniently erased my crutches. There seemed no way to fit them into the narrative.

I wasn't the only one for whom it was hard to fit together a disabled self and a movement identity. One of my fellow disability-rights activists, Kitty Cone, was arrested in her wheelchair at a civil rights sit-in in the early 1960s in Champaign, Illinois. After the local newspaper ran a picture of her on its front page, she received a piece of anonymous hate mail. The letter writer said that just because she was a "pathetic, ugly cripple" being "punished by God," she shouldn't try to force everyone to integrate with "niggers" who were "a baboon race." At the time only the racism struck her. Only years later did she realize the letter was as prejudiced about disability as it was about race.

A little while after we got off the bus, Faith and I saw the contingent of mustached men coming over the rise, chanting, carrying posters with the words "Avenge Che!" A few weeks before, Che Guevara had been killed in Bolivia, where he had gone in the hopes of leading a rebel uprising. Did the posters show the now-familiar portrait, which had been taken in 1960 at a protest rally, after a Belgian freighter carrying arms to Cuba had been blown up in Havana harbor, killing more than a hundred dock workers? While the original photograph showed the beginnings of crow's-feet around his eyes and the wispiness of his beard and mustache, the silk-screened rendering did away with the inevitable contours and roughness of any human face, turning him into an icon, without halftones or shading. Now when I think of that contingent coming over the rise, I see their ultraleft posturing, their machismo—for they were nearly all men—but at the time they had seemed to me to be priests of some higher order I could only aspire to enter. Of course I didn't know that in the diary Guevara had kept in Bolivia he had written often about his own disabling asthma: "Asthma is threatening me seriously and there is very little medicine in reserve. . . . My asthma continues getting worse and now I cannot sleep well. . . . I have asthma which I do not know how to stop. . . ."

And then people were handing us mimeographed leaflets with some lines wavering where the stencil had gone slightly askew against the platens of the machines—leaflets that weren't directed to the broader world but internally to the Left. Perhaps one of them had a hammer and sickle imposed over a five-pointed star, and the headline Build a Revolutionary, Anti-Imperialist Movement! From somewhere in the distance came the the haunting, reedy sound of bagpipes—anything goes!—played by one of the demonstrators. A man made his way through the demonstration toward me. I had met him at a weeklong movement school that kicked off Vietnam Summer, a project that was modeled on the Freedom Summer project of a few years before, which had sent college students to the South to organize voter registration drives. Plainly happy to see me again, he suggested that I come and march with his contingent. I realize now that he was interested in me. Did I realize it at the time? Did I not join him because he seemed not cool—slightly pudgy, wearing a plaid shirt? Or was I just frightened of any men who exhibited interest in me, my fear of my father having been generalized to all men?

As always there was a long period of waiting around at the start of the march, while everyone assembled and grouped themselves. And then, at last, we took off, lifting up signs that said NO VIET CONG EVER CALLED ME NIGGER, PEACE, END THE WAR, VICTORY TO THE NLF, IMMEDIATE WITHDRAWAL; Americans flags and National Liberation Front flags fluttered in the wind. Were there signs that said NEGOTIATE NOW? There must have been, carried by a few hardy souls who prided themselves on their moderation and sense of realpolitik.

And then, in my next memory, I was walking toward the Pentagon, walking so slowly that I drifted back from the rest of the Rhode Island contingent and ended up walking by myself, eventually finding myself underneath the banners and signs of Youth Against War and Fascism. I was embarrassed to be seen with them—they were a grouplet that had adopted wholesale the language of the left of thirty years ago. Faith must have gone off to march with a contingent of other black people. Her not wanting to be with a white person on certain occasions was one of those rules I understood, just as I understood that calling my white friends' parents by their first names made them feel hip, while it was unthinkable to do the same to the mothers and fathers of my black friends—a reminder of days in the South when all black people, no matter how prominent, would be addressed by their first names.

Then even the Youth Against War and Fascism contingent moved on ahead of me, and I was a straggler, bringing up the rear of the march.

In the next snapshot, I am at the Pentagon, but well back from the front lines, as I had promised my parents I would be. Despite all my wild posturings, I must have been scared myself, because I wouldn't have hesitated to break my promise to them if I had felt impelled to do so. Megaphones were calling out that people were being beaten and teargassed ahead of us. I remember—another of those snapshots—a man with a lock of hair falling over his forehead, running back to get water for those at the front to soak bandannas with, to alleviate the effects of the tear gas.

My next memory is being with Faith and Dawn and Mrs. Souza, walking by a line of troops, looking insectlike behind the rubber snouts of their gas masks, while Mrs. Souza looked steadfastly at the black men among them: "Brothers, what are you doing fighting for the man?" "Hey, brother! You're on the wrong side there. Come on over and be with your people." We could not see their faces, but I was sure they were frozen in shame.

A few weeks later someone stopped me in the hallway, told me to come into the school library: "You're in *Life* magazine!" There he showed me the magazine editorial, "Honest Dissent vs. Ugly Disorder," which warned about the growing "harsh tones" of the antiwar movement. It spoke of the "mainly sincere young demonstrators who had traveled long miles to oppose what many considered an evil foreign policy. Among them were the best—the young woman who by excruciating coordination managed to move from the Lincoln Memorial to the Pentagon on aluminum braces"—and went on to contrast the icon they'd turned me into with "hoodlums who spat on the troops, threw rocks through Pentagon windows, daubed the walls with lavatory obscenities."

I was, I have to say, flattered at the attention—there I was, singled out, me, Me, ME! But there was something about it that made me queasy, too. I couldn't have fully articulated what was wrong with turning me into a figure of rectitude on the basis of my disability. But somewhere inside me I understood that the whole thing was a bad bargain.

I became flattened. All the mixed emotions of that day—the drowsy daydreams, the sense of longing when I saw the chanting demonstrators coming over the rise with their posters of Che, the way I felt so cool when

Mrs. Souza called out the black soldiers—had disappeared as I was turned into a figure of easy nobility. Because I walked on crutches, I was assumed to be not just sincere, and not just in accord with the writer's views on what constituted the proper way to protest the war, but bordering on saintly, a representative of all that was good and ardent and pure and true.

It was probably harder for me to make that walk between the Lincoln Memorial and the Pentagon than for most of the demonstrators, but there may well have been other marchers with invisible disabilities—people with arthritis or heart conditions—for whom the walk was equally difficult. My crutches were stigmata, outer marks of an inner state. Furthermore, a year previously, I'd been in a group that had taken part in just the sort of action of which the editorial disapproved. In November 1966 Gen. Earle G. Wheeler, the chairman of the Joint Chiefs of Staff, had been scheduled to speak at Brown. A walkout and picket had been planned, but we wanted to do something more militant. About ten days before, Secretary of Defense Robert S. McNamara had spoken at Harvard. Members of Students for a Democratic Society had confronted him, some of them lying down in front of the wheels of his car. They'd demanded that he emerge for a debate; he came out and offered to answer "two questions," one of which was about how many South Vietnamese casualties there had been. McNamara—as anyone who has seen Errol Morris's *Fog of War* knows—had a statistician's mind and began to reel off the numbers of South Vietnamese military casualties. The demonstrators had been asking about the far more numerous civilian casualties, and jeered him down. A flying wedge of policemen had finally freed McNamara from the crowd, and he was led away through underground steam tunnels. One of the members of our antiwar crowd who had been at Brown but was now doing his graduate work at Harvard had taken part in that confrontation with McNamara, and it was partly as a result of his prompting that we decided to engage in a similar confrontation with General Wheeler.

General Wheeler addressed a noisy crowd of both pro- and antiwar sentiment, although the latter predominated. Pickets marched outside, and a contingent walked out when Wheeler began to speak. The newspaper the next day reported that "In a question-and-answer period after his talk, General Wheeler was asked hostile questions such as 'Please rationalize use of napalm on human beings in Viet Nam.' . . . General Wheeler replied that napalm 'is a condition of war in Viet Nam, just as rifle bullets are.' The rest of his answer was drowned out by hissing and booing from the audience." And then, as Wheeler's talk was about to finish, we rushed onto the stage. There were not enough of us, though, to surround him. Wheeler was hustled off the stage, and one of our group grabbed the microphone and made an antiwar statement. Campus police arrested one of our group.

I'm made into a noble figure often. Recently I was doing my exercise routine, which involves using my love of shopping to motivate myself to wheel a mile or two. I was wheeling in my manual chair to a shop on Berkeley's Fourth Street to look at objects displayed in a setting that seems more museumlike than commercial. I came to a corner with a button that had to be pushed in order to get a walk signal. But it was unreachable from a wheelchair. I leaned as far as I could out of my chair, but I still couldn't reach it, and I had to tilt my chair up on one wheel, bracing myself with one hand on the pole, in order to hit the button. I was mad: This is Berkeley, for Christ's sake, crip capital of the world, where you are more likely to pass a person using a wheelchair on the street than you are to pass a man wearing a necktie.

A woman, waiting in her car for the red arrow to turn to green, stared and stared at me as I was doing this. I glared back at her. Usually this results in one of two things—some people look away quickly; the more sophisticated give their eyes an unfocused stare, pretending to be gazing into the middle distance and that I just happen to fall within their range of vision. But she did neither. She continued staring at me.

The wait for a green arrow and the wait for a signal to cross the street are long at this intersection. I made a "roll down the window" gesture to her, turning my hand in a circle in the air.

She rolled down her window, and I called over to her, "Would you please stop staring at me!"

"I was looking at you with admiration."

"I find admiration as oppressive as pity!" I called back, but it's hard to change entrenched ways of looking at the world in a shouted discourse across an intersection. She didn't get it, and giving me a wave and a cheery smile, she at last turned left.

As sociologist John B. Kelly has written, "We need to investigate disability inspiration as a form of propaganda that glosses over oppression while simultaneously reassuring normals about the superiority of their ways." After all, if the button to push for the walk signal hadn't been inaccessible, if I'd been able to hit the button without going through contortions, there would have been nothing to find admirable in my attempt to get to the other side of the street. If the organizers of the March on the Pentagon had acknowledged that disabled people might have been among those taking part, and provided transportation along the parade route, then my valor and nobility would have disappeared.

The editorial writer's attitude toward me wasn't so different from the way I thought about the peasants of Vietnam, heroically resisting U.S. aggression. Around the time of the Pentagon march, I had ordered a book of photographs I'd seen advertised in the *National Guardian,* and among the other things I did when I wasn't doing my geometry and French homework was to flip through that book and gaze at the pictures of the brave peasants of Vietnam. My heroicizing them was an act of dehumanization; it reduced them to stick figures of nobility and courage.

Do I still have that book? After decades of accumulating and carting around books, I've made a determined effort to cast off some of that ballast, trying to free myself from the notion that the weight of my bookshelves bears a one-to-one relationship with the weight of my intellect. I ride my stair lift downstairs, and there it is, on the wooden shelves from Ikea: *Vietnam! Vietnam!* I'm all prepared, when I open it, to sneer at my own sentimentalizing—the young Vietnamese women with determined looks on their faces, holding rifles; the gentle, peace-loving peasants riding atop their water buffalo, their enormous cone-shaped hats perched atop their heads.

I climb back on the stair lift, holding the button with my left index finger, and flipping open the book as I begin the slow glide from the bottom of my loft to my study at the top. And sure enough, there were the women with rifles and determined looks on their faces, the peaceful peasants with their water buffaloes, and a photograph of U.S. Marines—boy-giants— leading blindfolded Vietnamese men away for questioning. The Vietnamese men so tiny they almost seem to belong to another species, a cousin to our gross, overfed American race. A photograph of a barefoot Vietnamese woman and a U.S. soldier standing amid rubble; he has a rifle pointed at her, her hands are folded in front of her face, perhaps in supplication, perhaps in despair. An elderly Vietnamese man with a white beard, blindfolded, gagged, tagged.

The horror of the war comes back to me, washes over me. My finger comes off the button, the stair lift stops, and suspended between upstairs and down, I start to sob.

SCHOOL HOUSE CANDY

At the age of sixteen I applied for a job at School House Candy in Paw-tucket, Rhode Island. Although I had earned money babysitting, I had never held a real job. I was paid only fifty cents an hour, but since Susan worked at Trinity Square, I often babysat for the actors. On a Friday or Saturday night, they'd go out after the performance, not coming home un-til two or three in the morning. The kids would have been sound asleep for hours and hours then, and I'd have been getting paid while I did my homework—occasionally—or read books, listened to music, smoked dope, watched TV, or slept—once, I dropped acid while I was babysitting, so I even got paid for tripping.

I'd make more than three times as much working in a factory, but even more important was that factory work was a real job, the sort where you knew from week to week the hours you were going to be working and the money you were going to earn. You had to provide your employer with a Social Security number. You could say to friends, "I've got to go to work," or "I get off work at six."

Every teenager in the Providence area in the 1960s seemed to have worked at School House Candy—even if only for a week or two. Perhaps there were jobs in the hidden recesses of the factory that required skills—mixing the chemicals and sugars and starches that went into the candy, maintaining adequate stocks of these ingredients—but the jobs high school kids got could be learned within minutes. Probably the newer you were at the job, the more efficient you were—you had not yet been demoralized by boredom nor had you figured out how to goof off while seeming to work. The pay was the minimum wage—$1.60 an hour.

School House Candy was located in one of the many brick buildings, vast and square, that dotted the landscape of Providence and Central Falls and Pawtucket. The red of their bricks had been muted by the layers of soot and grime that had accumulated over the decades. Their windows, too, seemed as if they had never been washed other than by rain, and were speckled with brown dirt. I imagine that this building—like most of the others—must once have been a textile mill, but the textile companies had all moved south, not just closer to where cotton was grown but farther away from the unionized workforces of the Northeast. By the late 1960s the former mills largely stood abandoned or had become factories where cheap costume jewelry was produced. A few others housed companies like School House Candy.

Working there was a rite of passage, an initiation into the world of work. From School House Candy one could move up to being a stringer, carder, or foot-press operator at one of the jewelry factories. My friends and my oldest sister described the scene to me. Down an endlessly turning conveyer belt would flow a river of one type of candy, perhaps lemon yellow lollipops— yellow lollipops, yellow lollipops, yellow lollipops, yellow lollipops, yellow lollipops, yellow lollipops. You stared at those yellow lollipops and thought you could never in your life be as sick of anything as you were of the sight of yellow lollipops. And then you would see that the yellow lollipops had been replaced by red lollipops. At first there would be relief. Something different to look at! And then, after a few minutes of watching red lollipops, red lol- lipops, red lollipops, red lollipops, red lollipops, red lollipops, red lollipops coming down the conveyor belt, you would find yourself longing to see something else, anything else—even a yellow lollipop.

Sometimes what came along the belt were Easter chicks, made of white marshmallow coated in yellow, three of which were to be placed on a white card and then sent on down the belt, where they would have black dots, representing their eyes, added to them. Farther down the belt they would be wrapped in plastic and the plastic sealed on both ends. They floated on down to the end of the line, where they were loaded into boxes, the boxes into cardboard cartons, ready for shipment. Sometimes the line flowed with other seasonal products, marshmallow Easter rabbits, ersatz chocolate jack-o'-lanterns, candy canes, hard candies in the shapes of Santa or reindeer or stars. Perhaps the candy was filled with preservatives, or perhaps the lack of any natural ingredients meant there was no possibility of deterioration. At any rate the lead time between the manufacturing of the candy and the holiday on which it was meant to be consumed was generally six months.

One day in July or August, a day when the temperature outside was in the nineties, and it must have been even hotter inside School House Candy, my sister Sandra came home from working there in a mood that mixed depression and fury, bemoaning the endless yellow marshmallow Easter chicks that had flowed along the belt that day, the sickly sweet smell of which clung to her hair and skin. I was in the bathtub when she got home, and she screamed at me, "Get out of the goddamn tub! I am so fucking hot! I need a bath! Let me in the goddamn bathroom!"

Who bought those cheap candies? Even when I was a kid and had a palate that could politely be described as undiscriminating, I hated the sort of candy produced there. Its only salient feature was its sugariness, and it had too much of that. After a few bites of it, the cloying sweetness would make your throat sore. I suppose the candy was bought by people who had so little money they could afford nothing else, or those who felt forced to go along with the rites of Halloween, and grudgingly gave out the fake chocolate jack-o'-lanterns or witches' hats made of artificially flavored black licorice.

I applied for a job at School House Candy, dutifully filling out the application. When I got ushered into the office for the interview, the man behind the desk was clearly embarrassed by my presence. When I try to call up the scene now, I cannot see his face, just a shiny suit of Dacron or Orlon, a no-wrinkle, drip-dry polyester shirt that had taken on a grayish sheen; a narrow necktie. He fiddled awkwardly with that narrow necktie, moving it back and forth between his index and middle fingers while he struggled to put together a coherent sentence. "Well, you know," he said. He glanced up at the ceiling. "Your . . . your . . . you know . . ." He stopped staring at the ceiling and stared at a point above my head. "Leg," he finally managed to say. "Leg."

Then he said the word "Insurance," and then, once again, he said, "Insurance. The thing is," and at last he seemed able to speak, "the insurance company worries about these things. I would have to talk to them and get an okay from them."

He told me he would check with the insurance company and call me back, and I actually believed him.

But of course he didn't call me.

In the mid-1950s Hugh Gallagher, who had been disabled as a result of polio, seeking to fulfill a lifelong dream of attending Oxford, applied for a Rhodes Fellowship. Gallagher's application was neither accepted nor rejected. It was simply returned to him unprocessed. When Cecil Rhodes established the fellowships, he had stipulated that they were to go to those who were "fit in mind and body." Gallagher later learned that a special meeting had been convened to decide what to do about his application. The decision was made to act as if the application had never been received. Gallagher refers to this as a "very English sort of rejection," but to me it seemed the way that disability discrimination often happened—obliquely, with an air of embarrassment and averted glances, the word "uh" punctuating the conversation.

How often I have experienced what I did with the man at School House Candy, who could not put a sentence together. In the face of disability, language itself becomes crippled. It trips over itself, it stutters, it becomes awkward, ungainly, even paralyzed. A little while ago my friend Susan, who had just come back from visiting her parents told me that her mother asked after me—although not by name. "What did she say?" I asked. "How's your friend with the funny last name—Hand? Toe?" "No," Susan said. "That's not how she described you." "Oh," I said, drawing the word out and laughing. "How's your disabled friend?" No, not that. "*Handicapped?*" I asked. "Crippled?" It turned out that Susan's mother had said, "How's your friend who's—uh—uh?"

When I started writing fiction, dialogue came easily to me—I think because I was used to listening for what people were saying beneath their words. All my life I've had to understand how utterances sought to conceal as well as to reveal—and yet, inevitably, showed the very thing their speakers thought they were hiding. I had to finely hone my ability to hear what was beneath polite lies and evasions, to see the discomfort that people thought they were keeping secret.

I didn't argue with the man at School House Candy, or with any of the other people who out-and-out refused to hire me because of my disability.

Having spent the day writing about School House Candy, I meet a friend for dinner. Pepper asks me how my day was, and I tell him I've been writing about work, about not getting hired at School House Candy, about the yellow lollipops and the Easter marshmallow chicks—he remembers those, and shudders—and the red lollipops, and the summer heat in the unair-conditioned factory.

"Honey, did you *really* want to work there?" he asks, laughing.

Well, yes, I did. And it wasn't just that I needed the money, although I did need the money.

Getting out of working at School House Candy was a bit like getting out of gym class. All the other girls complained about gym: about the uniforms—ridiculous blue outfits with bloomers, something our mother might have worn in the 1930s; about the showers where the water was always too cold; about the gym teacher who kept a logbook to record their menstrual periods—girls were excused from gym when they had their periods. I only heard exasperated reports from other students, about how she had accused them of faking, booming out so that everyone could hear: "You just had your period three weeks ago!" Or she might shout out a girl's name, adding, "You haven't had your period in five weeks. There's nothing *wrong*, is there?"

I could believe anything about the gym teacher, since once a week, in the time slot usually reserved for gym, she taught a class called "Health and Hygiene," which I did have to attend. When the subject was dental health, she had talked at length about her own dental work, telling us proudly that she had solid gold fillings, far superior to the ordinary amalgam generally used. She had then walked up and down the rows between the desks, her right index finger hooked into her open mouth, so that we could each in turn gaze into her mouth and see her dental work for ourselves. Another time she told us about a crippled beggar in Mexico who had asked her for money. Instead of giving him pesos, she had given him a lecture—it was impossible to imagine that she had deigned to speak in a language other than God's own English—about laziness and malingering, and at the end of her lecture he had gotten up and walked! Oh, there was nothing really wrong with him—what these people needed was just a good strong admonition to pull themselves up by their bootstraps.

Did I want my own fusty gym uniform? Did I want the gym teacher to shout at me that I got my period too often? Did I want to work at School House Candy and come home at the end of the day sweaty and exhausted and nauseated? Yes, I did. I wanted that chance, to complain and moan and hate along with everyone else.

I was not, of course, asking for what we would today call "reasonable accommodation" at School House Candy—for instance, a job that could be done seated, or even a stool on which I could perch while working on the line. Such a notion was unimaginable in those days. I applied for the job fully expecting to stand for my entire shift. Would I have been in pain at the end of a shift? Of course I would have been.

I did not know that anyone else had ever experienced the rejection and discrimination I was experiencing. I must have heard of Randolph Bourne, an opponent of World War I, whose book *Youth and Life* was considered the original manifesto of the youth counterculture. And I had read John Dos Passos's sprawling trilogy, *USA*, in which Bourne was described as "a tiny twisted unscared ghost in a black cloak hopping along the grimy old brick and brownstone streets still left in downtown New York, crying out in a shrill soundless giggle: War is the health of the state." Had I realized that the words "tiny," "twisted," "hopping" were Dos Passos's way of describing Bourne's disability—a facial deformity stemming from a "messy birth" and a hunched back caused by tuberculosis of the spine?

In his seminal essay, "The Handicapped," published in the *Atlantic Monthly* in 1911, Bourne wrote of his quest for work:

I besieged for nearly two years firm after firm, in search of a permanent position, trying everything in New York in which I thought I had the slightest chance of success, meanwhile making a precarious living from a few music lessons. The attitude toward me ranged from "You can't expect us to create a place for you," to, "How could it enter your head that we should find any use for a man like you?"

With his family in straitened circumstances, Bourne's need for work was acute:

There is a poignant mental torture that comes with such an experience—the urgent need, the repeated failure, or rather the repeated failure even to obtain a chance to fail, the realization that those at home can ill afford to have you idle, the growing dread of encountering people—all this is something that those who have never been through it can never realize.

I didn't know that Randolph Bourne had been through what I was going through. I had read a lot about the Free Speech Movement at the University of California at Berkeley in 1964—credited with being the big bang that started the student movement. Had I read of Jacobus tenBroek, a leading faculty supporter of that movement? If I had read anything about him, I would almost certainly have known that he was blind, since any description of him would have highlighted this point. I wouldn't have known that he had cowritten a text, *Hope Deferred: Public Welfare and the Blind,* in which he spoke of the restrictions on the lives of blind people as a civil rights issue.

I didn't know that in New York in the 1930s, a group of disabled workers and would-be workers—many of whom had, in all likelihood, been paralyzed by polio in the 1916 New York City epidemic—found themselves deemed, by Roosevelt's Works Progress Administration, as "unemployable." They had organized as the League of the Physically Handicapped to protest such discrimination.

Sylvia Bassoff, one of the organizers, spoke of her experiences before she joined the group: "Well, I found I couldn't get a job. Not because there was a Depression. I found I couldn't get a job because I was handicapped." She enrolled at a business school, and became a whiz at taking dictation and typing. "In my naïveté, I figured, 'I'll graduate from the Drake Business School and they're all going to grab me.' . . . Well, nobody grabbed me. . . . Some people who . . . got jobs . . . didn't begin to be as good as I was." Unable to get work in the private sector, she was humiliated at being forced to turn to a sheltered workshop run by the Brooklyn Bureau of Charities, where she was paid $3.50 for every thousand envelopes she addressed by hand. When a member of the league told her that it was organizing to get jobs for people with disabilities, Sylvia said, "Jobs? Anything to get out of here."

The early members of the league had more in common than their identity as "the handicapped." They were largely Jewish, from working-class families, the children of recent immigrants from eastern and southern Europe. Not only had they come from backgrounds in which education was highly regarded and the work ethic strong, they shared a radical political outlook. Coming from families and communities in which leftist ideology was predominant, they were used to thinking of social, rather than individual, solutions to problems. But while the New York Left—in which many of them had their roots—embraced their cause, they often did so in a way that further stigmatized people with disabilities. When the league was picketing the WPA, the *Daily Worker* described them as "dragging their own lame bodies back and forth," bodies "twisted by infantile paralysis." At other times they were described as "paralysis victims" or "helpless crippled people." A headline in the *Daily Worker* played on pity when it declared "Brave LaGuardia Police Beat, Club, Jail Crippled Jobless."

Shortly after Roosevelt himself became disabled, a friend of his mother's asked, "Now [that] he is a cripple, will he ever be anything else?" Roosevelt was to spend the next decade of his life cobbling together an answer to that question—at first by trying to "unmake" himself as a cripple; later by creating the story of himself as a man who, through personal heroism and grit, had "overcome" his disability. And yet, when Roosevelt spoke of the necessity of creating jobs for the unemployed rather than simply giving them money, saying, "To dole out relief is to administer a narcotic, a subtle destroyer of the human spirit. . . . We must preserve not only the bodies of the unemployed from destitution but also their self-respect," his words reflect the experience he had finding his social identity taken from him in the wake of his disability. How ironic that these workers were being deemed unemployable by an administration headed by a president who would himself have been deemed unemployable by his own administration's regulations!

No doubt many of those who had formed the League of the Physically Handicapped found employment during World War II, when labor shortages brought millions of people into well-paying employment: Rosie the Riveter is a familiar figure; so too is the history of the great internal migration, as black sharecroppers and tenant farmers moved from the South to war-industry employment in Detroit, Oakland, and Chicago. People with disabilities also gained entry into the workforce during the war. Robert Huse found work at Raytheon during that time; his coworkers were women who had never been in the paid workforce before, men too old for military service, and other disabled people. Employment did not mean accommodation, however: Huse got to work half an hour early so that if he couldn't find a parking space close to the front door he would have time to hike across the parking lot. He noticed that others of his disabled coworkers were doing the same, and put a note in the company suggestion box: Why not set some parking spaces aside at the front for disabled workers? (It was never acted upon.) While wartime employment brought something of a reprieve from discrimination, it also brought with it the knowledge that what had been gained could be lost. When the war ended, would things go back to being as they had been before?

Huse had a coworker at Raytheon, a man with an amputated leg, who was also an alcoholic and had gotten fired for poor work. Later Huse saw him on the street in Boston:

> His hair had turned almost white and came down over his ears. He was unshaven and filthy. Fanned out in his hands were several pencils and beside him was a battered pie pan, which held several coins. . . . "Take a good look, kid, because this is what happens to us." That night, Huse had a nightmare that he was penniless and hungry, and searching for a street corner on which to sell his pencils. "On every corner the one-legged man sits and leers at me, I hurry by. His voice follows me, 'You'll be back, kid, you'll be back . . .' "

If I had not been so mired in contempt for other people with disabilities, I might have talked to those around me who were similarly situated: a man who was part of the local civil rights movement and had cerebral palsy; a boy who also attended my high school, who had also had polio and walked on wooden crutches, toward whom I felt an almost physical repulsion.

Oh, the contempt I felt for my high school classmate! I do not remember his name, and I cannot recall anything about his face. What I do remember are those old-fashioned wooden crutches, which splayed out from his body. Pieces of foam rubber covered the tops of the crutches, where they were tucked under his arms, and also covered the grips. The sweat from his underarms and hands sank into that foam rubber, leaving them with a musty smell and a sunk-in grittiness that could not be washed away. (I knew both the smell and the grittiness, because I had once had such crutches.) My crutches were aluminum, and I had replaced the gray hand grips they had come with with brightly colored ones designed for a kid's bicycle, with red and pink streamers coming from them.

It was vitally important to me that I not be seen with the other boy who had had polio. (I could make up a name for him, but let me leave that gaping hole of the name I don't remember.) People might think we were two of life's rejects, clinging to each other: or worse, they might think our companionship sweet, touching, poignant, and above all fitting.

I told myself I had good reason for my contempt. I did not hate him because he was disabled. I hated him because his shirt was always untucked. I had contempt for him because his mother picked him up after school—he was a spoiled baby.

My mother did not pick me up after school. I used to walk, along with everyone else, from the rise on the far edge of downtown Providence across the pedestrian mall—designed to make the experience of shopping there more like a visit to the suburban shopping centers that were springing up in Warwick and Cranston—to wait for the 52 Hope bus that would drop me at the corner of Hope and Larch Streets; from there I would walk two and a half blocks up the hill, passing Catalpa Road and Ivy Street and then letting myself in the back door of our house, so exhausted that I would throw my crutches and coat onto the living room floor and collapse on the couch.

The backpack had not yet become a common item—it was then used almost exclusively by hikers and the military—and so I carried my books in the green canvas bookbag my mother—like all Cliffies—had used at Radcliffe. I couldn't, of course, carry it the way she had, her hand holding the loop and the bag resting on her back, since each of my hands was holding a crutch. I put the loop of the bookbag over my left shoulder and, as I swayed back and forth as I walked, the bookbag banged first against my crutch, then against my body, a metronome keeping its own off-kilter beat. Inside the bag were my textbooks—Ancient History and English, Latin I—year after year, Latin I, as I kept failing the class.

I then waited at the bus stop with everyone else, clambered onto the bus with everyone else, dropped my dime—or was it thirty-five cents?—into the fare box. It was at this bus stop that a drunken man had approached me and muttered an incomprehensible question. I dutifully said, as my mother had taught me, "Excuse me?" He repeated his mumbled question: Was he asking me if the bus was going to be late? "I don't know," I said. A few seconds after I had answered him, I was mortified to realize that what he had asked me was, "Do you want to get laid?"

If I hadn't been so fearful of other disabled people, I might have asked them how they had negotiated the surprisingly perilous journey into the world of work. They might have been able to suggest some strategies to me—or we might at least have been able to commiserate. And if I had not been so intent on protecting my parents from the effects of my disability, I might have talked to them.

But, like the man at School House Candy, embarrassed by my very presence as a job seeker, I, too, found myself unable to articulate a clean sentence. The words to describe what I was experiencing came to me singly, in isolation—"discrimination" . . . "unfair"—along with a sense of shame that I could not name even to myself, never mind to anyone else. The ideas that would become fully formed with the disability-rights movement were now feelings, sensations within my body; scattered, disconnected words, a sudden gust of shame that expressed itself as me hanging my head, cringing. I had a sense that my problem was a social one, not an individual one—but, having cut myself off from other disabled people, and knowing nothing of what those who had gone before me had experienced, I was unable to translate that vague sensibility into anything else. In short, I lacked both a history and a community.

After a few more experiences such as I had had at School House Candy, I called the Rhode Island Department of Vocational Rehabilitation—Voc Rehab for short—because it seemed that they should be able to help me. The man on the other end of the line explained that they would be glad to evaluate me, to give me a battery of tests, to train me for a job, but no, they could do nothing about helping me find a job, and no, they knew of no places that would be willing to consider hiring me. "Training," he said again. "Training." The word made me think of Mr. Popper's trained penguins in a book my mother had read to us as children; it made me think of special-ed classes, which in those days were divided into those for the "educable mentally retarded" and the "trainable mentally retarded," "trainable" being the lesser of the two. I wasn't retarded, I wasn't a penguin, I did not want to be "trained" for anything. Did I argue with him?

Did I say, "What's the point in training us if no one will hire us?" I don't think I did. I think I muttered, "Thank you," and hung up.

I ended up going back to babysitting. At thirteen I had felt thrilled to be left alone in a near-stranger's house: to play their records and snoop through their drawers, to leaf through their books looking for dirty ones—which one could immediately spot in those days: The Supreme Court had decided that material could only be considered obscene if it both aroused "prurient interest" and was utterly without "redeeming social value." Without fail, dirty books had an introduction written by a physician or psychologist setting forth why the material one was about to read had the necessary "redeeming social value." But at sixteen I was no longer thrilled at being left alone in a grown-up's house; snooping had lost its appeal, as had reading dirty books. I was more than ready to move on.

LONDON

My senior year of high school, I sent away for college applications—mostly from the schools that, as the sixties drew to a close, had inaugurated programs they trumpeted as being "open" and "experimental." Throughout the last three years of high school, my grades had ranged wildly: A's in English and history, F's in math and Latin. I took Algebra I twice, Geometry I twice, Latin I three times. My SAT scores were high but not spectacular. I knew that getting accepted at a college was going to involve finding someplace willing to take a gamble on my offbeat history, my apparent maturity, and my promise.

I never got around to finishing the applications. I filled out the easy sections, noting my name and address, the date and place of my birth, and answered the questions about physical handicap that were then standard, but I kept putting off writing the essays, getting my transcripts sent. The deadlines passed with the half-completed pages shoved in a desk drawer. With my peculiar mix of indolence and wildness, I decided to take a year off and go to Europe.

Just before the end of my senior year, I moved out of my parents' house to an apartment I shared with another young woman, splitting the rent of fifty dollars a month. I set about trying to find a job, enduring that old round of rejections.

I couldn't afford the thirty-five cents for the bus fare the day I had an interview at the phone company, so I walked the mile from our apartment. It had been years since I'd worn clunky orthopedic shoes, but it was nearly impossible to find regular shoes that would fit my misshapen feet. The medical word used to describe my right foot is "equine," suggesting a resemblance to a horse's hoof. The lack of muscle function in my foot means that my toes have, over the years, slowly curled downward and inward, as has the foot itself, almost like the bound feet Chinese women once had. Unshod, my feet never hurt, but with shoes on, they often do. Once a friend who has spina bifida told me she had no sensation in her feet. "Oh," I said. "No sensation in your feet. That sounds like heaven on earth to me!" During the course of my walk to the phone company, the Band-Aids I'd applied on top of the blisters rubbed off, and blood and pus seeped down my right heel.

After I filled out the application, which had been handed to me by the receptionist, the woman in personnel came out. She looked at my crutches and said, "I'm sorry. You wouldn't be able to get around well enough to work here." Did I say anything at all back to her? I think maybe I said, "Really, I can get around pretty well." "I'm sorry," she said. Her tone of voice suggested that she was both sorry I'd had polio, and sorry that I didn't understand the rules of the game better and had had the temerity to apply for a job. Why didn't I argue with her? Or at least tell her that I'd walked a mile to get there? Was it shame? Was it the way I'd been taught always to make other people feel comfortable about my disability? Or knowing that arguing wasn't going to do any good? Probably all of those.

Finally I got a job as an editorial assistant at the American Mathematical Society because I was friends with the son of the society's director. The American Mathematical Society published books and journals, filled with phrases like "semisimple involutory Hopf algebra," "nonreal zero," "piecewise linear groups," "vector bundles," "the Neumann problem," "knot theory," "topological quantum field theories." One did not have to know anything about mathematics in order to do mathematical proofreading. My job was merely to make certain that the printed copy matched the original typescript. In a soundproof booth, I would sit opposite another editorial assistant, one of us reading aloud from the long galleys of the typeset text and the other one following along on the manuscript the author had submitted. Once or twice I was able to follow something of the articles that I read—an introductory sentence, perhaps. But most of it was incomprehensible. The sentence, "Let β be a one-one Hilbert-Schmidt operator on H and e_1, e_2, e_3 . . . be an orthonomal basis for H," would be read aloud as, "Cap-L-let-beta-be-a-one-hyphone-cap-H-Hilbert (h-i-l-b-e-r-t) hyph-cap-S-Schmidt (s-c-h-m-i-d-t)-operator-on-cap-H-underscored-and-small-e-sub-one-com-small-e-sub-2-com-small-e-sub-three-three-ellipsis-be-an-orthonormal-basis-for-cap-H-point," the words spat out at a terrific rate. Those Dada sentences would be followed by absurdist equations. At night when I lay down to sleep, my brain would generate meaningless equations from the day's detritus: An enormous Σ raised to the infinite power equal to an A added to a P, enclosed within parentheses and squared, would drift in front of me; it would disappear to be followed by another equally meaningless equation. Perhaps the equations weren't meaningless: Maybe like that monkey eternally plonking the keys of a typewriter, I conjured an equation that made sense. I might even have assembled an equation that solved one of the seemingly insoluble riddles of mathematics, although I would never have known that I had done so.

The worst part of the job was that I lost my ability to read for pleasure. If I picked up *Moby-Dick*, I couldn't read the opening sentences as "Call me Ishmael. Some years ago—never mind how long precisely—having little or no money in my purse, and nothing particular to interest me on shore, I thought I would sail about a little and see the watery part of the world." Instead that sentence would tumble through my brain as "Cap-C-Call-me-cap-I-Ishmael-point-cap-S-Some-years-ago-single-em dash-never-mind-how-long-precisely-single-em-dash-having-little-or-no-money-in-my-purse-com-and-nothing-particular-to-interest-me-on-shore-com-cap-I-thought-cap-I-would-sail-about-a-little-and-see-the-watery-part-of-the-world-point."

My job was eight hours of drudgery through which I dragged myself, but I saved two-thirds of the paycheck I got every month—my parents' training in frugality stood me in good stead. After six months I'd saved enough to buy a one-way ticket on Icelandic Airways, which offered rock-bottom prices on flights from New York to Brussels, with a stopover in Reykjavík. After that my plans were vague: I'd travel and be back to the States in September, maybe move to New York and take classes at The New School.

But as summer gave way to fall, and my classmates headed off to college, I sank into one of those grim spells of depression that had plagued me throughout my life.

———

I had planned to take the Greyhound bus from Providence and then a second bus to Kennedy Airport in New York to catch my flight on Icelandic, but a few days before I was due to leave, it turned out that my father also had to fly out of New York for a meeting, and since my mother was going to give him a ride there, I also got a ride. We dropped my father off first. He had kissed my mother good-bye and was starting to saunter away when she called after him, "Jack! You forgot to say good-bye to Anne!" He came back as I was clambering out of the backseat into the front, and gave me a boozy peck on the cheek.

As the plane rose, I could feel my depression leaving me, a caul of sadness tearing away as the plane soared upward.

From Brussels I took a bus to Paris. We drove through French towns, and I was surprised to see the flat stone fronts of the houses meeting the sidewalk. Had I really assumed that houses in Europe would look like those in America, set in the middle of square yards surrounded by picket fences? I suppose I must have.

And what else do I remember from that bus trip? The face of a man who sat in front of me, who reminded me of Jimmy, the first man I had loved. All the solid things I have forgotten—the names of housemates, the addresses of flats and apartments where I once lived, those Latin conjugations and declensions I spent hours memorizing—all those forgotten and then the ephemeral things that have stayed, like the face of the man whose name I never even knew.

He was in his mid-thirties (old, so old!), with a sallow complexion—the sort of face that looks grizzled if it isn't shaved twice a day. His skin had the waxy quality of someone who sweats a lot, and I could picture a handkerchief in his pocket, with which he would dab the perspiration from his brow, which would retain, even after many washings, an umber cast. He was not so much short as compact. I was drawn to him, and he terrified me.

Could that Anne who was riding the bus between Brussels and Paris have articulated those words, "He terrified me?" I think not. I was in the grip of sensations that were inchoate, feelings I couldn't yet give shape to by cloaking them in words. I was a just-turned-eighteen-year-old, straddling the border between girlhood and womanhood, riding the bus between Brussels and Paris, with her crutches slid under the seat, carrying about within her a mass of contradictions, of things that couldn't be spoken, of histories that had been buried, tamped down. A girl-woman, at once so fearless and so afraid.

Did he offer me one of his unfiltered Gauloise? Perhaps. And perhaps I accepted it, inhaled the unfamiliar tobacco, tasting darker and mustier—more European, more grown-up than the lightly roasted American tobacco I was used to. Perhaps I got the tip of the cigarette wet with saliva and was vaguely embarrassed at having done so—the excess of saliva my mouth produced seemed evidence of my being too much, excessive, overflowing my boundaries. How the air on that bus must have filled up with clouds of cigarette smoke! In those days everyone's hair and clothes reeked of stale smoke, so omnipresent we didn't even notice it. When he pulled off his leather jacket, he released a reek of pure maleness.

After my father retired he went for months at a time without bathing or showering. I don't know why—maybe it was because he was depressed, and inattention to personal hygiene is a common symptom of depression, especially in the elderly. Or maybe it wasn't so much a symptom of depression but a way of broadcasting his despair, hoping that someone, anyone, would notice, as I had flunked my spelling tests in the seventh grade, flying the only distress signal I knew. Or maybe, as so often happened, my father's anger and sadness melded together. Maybe he was simultaneously mourning, and enraged at, the coming of old age, the loss of his status and powers, the prospect of death. And maybe his refusing to bathe was both an act of aggression and a refusal to be diminished: *You can't avoid me! You can't pretend I'm not in the room! Smell me! Smell my stink! Here I am!* and also a way of saying, "I'm dying! I'm dying! Can't you smell me rotting?"

During the period when my father wasn't bathing, my parents came to visit me in Detroit, where I was teaching creative writing at Wayne State University. Every time I came within a few feet of my father, his smell would hit me. He smelled the way a badly deteriorated homeless person smells. Sometimes, when I pass someone like that on the street, I instinctively pull my purse closer to me. Not out of any fear of being robbed, but because I want to pull closer those amulets I carry around with me—the twenties fresh from the cash machine, the credit cards imprinted not just with my name—which, after all, others may share—but with a number that is mine alone; the driver's license that proves who I am; the keys to my house, to my car. All those things that protect me from sinking into the state of being a sweaty, stinking animal, like that person I am passing. I have a home to go to with faucets that open up and pour out water, hot or cold, potions to wash away my smell. I have a closet full of clean clothes and a washing machine and dryer. I can roll into a store and buy myself new clothes, clothes that smell of nothing at all.

During my father's visit, I sank into depression. After weeks of stumbling through my days, feeling as if I had a rock in my chest where my heart should have been, I went to a therapist. During the course of that rambling first session: When had the depression started? About three weeks ago. What had been going on then? Well, a couple of things. A class in which I felt my students didn't appreciate me. The endless gray skies of a Detroit winter. And my parents had been visiting. That was hard. My father doesn't bathe, he smells awful.

"Smell is so visceral. It bypasses the more rational parts of the brain," the therapist said, and that spell of depression vanished as if a genie had snapped his fingers together.

Of course, on that day, late in December 1969, when I was riding the bus from Brussels to Paris, the old man my father would become didn't yet exist. My father was forty-nine, younger than I am now. Yet that future self existed somewhere inside him, as the woman I am now was nascent in that eighteen-year-old girl. I already knew his rage, the way he was never contained, his maleness; I was already frightened by the smell of him, so that the scent of a man would always stir in me a mix of fear and anger and longing, touch the gaping hole in my heart that was my love for my father.

In Paris I stayed in a hotel recommended in *Europe on $5 a Day*. The cheap rooms touted in that guidebook were all up in the garret, so after explaining to the desk clerk that I really did want the cheapest room, even if it was on the top floor, I climbed up five flights of stairs, dropped off my backpack in a tiny room with a narrow cot and a sink in the corner, and then walked down the stairs again, making my way to a corner café where the waiter, predictably, sneered at my attempts at French. By then I had already spent the daily allowance of five dollars I had allotted myself, and so I returned to my room alone. I lay on the narrow bed, reading a paperback book I had brought from home, telling myself over and over again, "I'm in Paris, I'm in Paris," trying to summon up the romance, the foreignness, the excitement I ought to feel. A mouse ran out from under my bed, stopped in the middle of the floor, and regarded me with a look of disdain.

I didn't last long in France—I couldn't take the unabashed Gallic stare. My second day in Paris I'd been humiliated when a whole class of French schoolboys, picturesque in their short pants and caps, had stopped in their tracks and gaped en masse at me as I moved through the Métro on my crutches.

I went to England, where, after all, they spoke English and were too polite to gawk openly. My fellow passengers on the Tube might stare at me, but they were covert stares—eyes peeking up above their newspapers, or gazing at me while my head was turned away. If I caught them, and glared back, they would be abashed—either looking away quickly or offering me a conciliatory smile.

I knocked around for a while, working without papers and sharing a flat with some other young women—although in those days we called ourselves girls.

With that same wild mix of passivity and risk taking that had impelled me to London in the first place, I married an Englishman.

I try to get back to my memories of that time, but I seem unable to form complete sentences. Instead scattered images and words flit into my mind: the name of the pub where we used to drink, the Bricklayer's Arms. Ben's face. A mauve maxidress I owned. But each of those images and words is draped in a mantle of shame. It's like walking into a beach house that's been shut up for the winter, furniture covered with sheets, so that the rough outline, the form of things can be seen—yes, over there's the sofa, the coffee table, the rocking chair—and yet everything remains indistinct, the textures, the fine particularities hidden.

But if I stare at those images, they become clearer. So I'll begin there, with the flat itself, a place of little light and less air. A long narrow corridor. Three rooms off that corridor, although we lived almost entirely in the front room, sleeping on the fold-out sofa there, listening to music, hanging out with our friends. The long narrow corridor ended in a refrigeratorless galley kitchen. Lack of a refrigerator, which back home meant you had slipped beneath the ranks of the poverty stricken into the ranks of the destitute, here marked you as unpretentious, ordinary. Beyond the kitchen was a rectangular patch of trash-filled ground referred to as the garden, although nothing deigned to grow there but a few rangy weeds. It seemed that even the wind-borne seeds of mugwort and dandelion had looked down on our backyard scrap of dirt and headed on somewhere more promising.

The long narrow corridor of our flat, with its floral print wallpaper that, I imagine, had once been bright yellow with red roses, although the colors had long since faded to ochre and a color that could charitably be described as salmon. Here and there around those once-red roses, living flowers of black were entwined: mold, which Londoners blithely described as "rising damp," and treated as a quite unremarkable and expected phenomenon, spread itself in floral patterns to form a smutty bouquet.

In that corridor—I was careful not to use the American word "hall"—Ben one day painted a black peace symbol, stretching from floor to ceiling, so that after that we had an ugly peace symbol on top of our even uglier wallpaper. And now that memory sparks a whole chain of associations: He painted that peace symbol so that anyone who ventured into our flat might know that, despite the appearance of things we were *political.* We might live in a dank and airless London flat with faded floral wallpaper, a flat that resembled the vast majority of other London flats. We might have in our kitchen an electric kettle and a teapot with a crocheted cosy, and a box of PG Tips tea; our kitchen cupboards might contain Weetabix, Horlicks, and Marmite (a foul concoction, made to be spread on bread, which the label said contained "extracts" of yeast and vegetables) along with a tin of Lyle's Golden Syrup with the drawing of bees buzzing around a lion's carcass and the biblical quote beneath it, "From the strong came forth sweetness." Our dustbin, like the dustbins of nearly all our neighbors, might contain a couple of crumpled pages from the *News of the World* or the *Evening Standard,* a splotch of grease spreading across the lurid headlines—MP LOVE NEST, IRA BOMB HORROR—in which our orders of cod or sole had been carried home from the fish-and-chips place up the road. We might drink our tea out of chipped white porcelain cups, decorated with sprigs of posies, the insides of which had a network of cracks stained brown by a lifetime's worth of tea—we had bought ours from the Oxfam Shop on the High Street, to which they must have been donated by the offspring of a woman lately deceased or taken into care.

We might have an electric fire fronted with a design of fake coals that glowed as if they were really burning—many Londoners were still nostalgic for the coal fires outlawed in the wake of London's killer fogs—a lethal mix of pollution and fog. In short, while our surroundings might suggest that we were quite ordinary, that eight-foot-diameter black peace symbol told a quite different story.

And from that memory, another one: a white friend we had whose nickname was Panther Mike, who was gaga over the black militant Angela Davis—crazy about her in the way that teenage girls can go mad for rock stars. His curly hair formed a halo around his head, a pale homage to her magnificent Afro. He used to pull out his wallet to show the picture of Davis he'd clipped from the newspaper, and exclaim over the gap between her two front teeth the way a proud papa points out an offspring's dimples or button nose.

Yes, and now from that one memory another one follows, and another. First of all the demonstration Ben and I, along with a few friends we had in common, went to in Trafalgar Square, a few days after we had met. I don't remember what the demonstration was about, whether it was against the war in Vietnam or apartheid. What I do remember was that I was in a crowd of demonstrators across the street from the square itself, when the police suddenly decided they wanted us to move. People linked arms, and I did, too, dangling my crutches from my forearms. We pushed back against the cops, who were pushing back against us, their truncheons gripped in front of them, shoving us back to the metal traffic barricades, cemented into the pavement, designed to keep pedestrians in their place. At American demonstrations I'd developed a good sense of when trouble was brewing and been able to get myself safely away, but here I hadn't foreseen that I was going to get caught in a confrontation. I was terrified that I was going to get knocked over, trampled by the crowd, and the two strangers on either side of me, with whom I'd ended up linking arms, saw my distress and began to call out, "Let her get out of here! She needs to get out of here!" The mutual shoving stopped for a minute, I was allowed to go free, and then it resumed.

When we were all together in someone's front room after the demonstration, Ben reprimanded me for wearing sandals. I should have worn closed-toe shoes. It was all in the context of a general rant he was carrying out against women at demonstrations—I think the actual word he used was "chicks"—and how we weren't tough enough. In my mind I responded to him: *It's not as easy as all that. It's almost impossible for me to find a pair of shoes that fit my feet, that I can walk in.* But I didn't actually speak those words. Partly I knew it was that any explanation of how a disabled body functions almost inevitably seems to trigger a series of questions masked as advice: Have you tried acupuncture/herbs/surgery/physical therapy/swimming/Reikki/yoga/aromatherapy/shiatsu/Chinese herbs? Have you been Rolfed? Or outright advice: You should go to Cuba/a homeopath/the Mayo Clinic/an Ayurvedic physician/Columbia Presbyterian/a naturopath. You should wear orthopedic shoes.

All of that is true but too easy. There was more to my silence on that day than my need to keep advice at bay. I was drawn to his slight air of contempt for me. It felt familiar.

When I look back on this scene—look back on it from the lofty perch on which I now sit, atop the passage of time and decades of psychotherapy—what glares out at me was his utter lack of concern for the fact that I had been caught in a dangerous situation, had almost been hurt. We weren't yet officially "in love," hadn't slept together yet, although we'd necked and were drawn to each other. Somewhere inside of me—some part of myself I couldn't see then but see so clearly now—I was relieved that he hadn't been scared for me, hadn't wanted to protect me, hadn't been concerned that I might have been hurt. Whatever longings I had to be comforted, to be watched out for, to be protected, to be taken care of, were buried deep inside me. To have known them would have threatened that fortress of independence and toughness I had built around myself.

More than anything else I didn't want to be pitied. I understood—I think I had known it from the time I was a very young child—that pity is always shadowed by contempt, and that those who pity can never really see the ones who are pitied; the act of pitying erases their individuality, turns them into objects. But that someone could show concern for me without pitying me, could worry about me without obliterating me—of that I had no experience.

We fell in love. We made love over and over again, sometimes four or five or six times a day. We smoked dope—not the American grass I was used to, which here was prized and rare, but gummy hashish, which was pulverized between thumb and forefinger and sprinkled over tobacco. We dropped acid together; occasionally we did speed. We ate sweet-and-sour pork from the Chinese place on the Upper Richmond Road and chicken vindaloo from the Indian take-out on the Lower Richmond Road, drank endless cups of milky, sugary tea. We went every night to the Bricklayer's Arms, which everyone called "the Brick"—at least on the nights we didn't go to a film—I never said "the movies" anymore, it was one of those American words, like "cookie," that could send my friends into gales of stoned laughter. At the Brick I drank Coke (I didn't like the taste of alcohol), and Ben drank pint after pint of bitter. We saw *Easy Rider* and *Five Easy Pieces* and a 1931 movie called *Five and Dime* with Marion Davies and Leslie Howard. We saw every film ever made by the great Russian film director Sergey Eisenstein—not just *Strike!* and *October* and *The Battleship Potemkin* and *Ivan the Terrible, Parts I and II*, but even the remains of one that had been destroyed on Stalin's orders, reconstructed from clips of film that had somehow survived, stills, a voice-over narrating portions of the script. We saw films by Hitchcock and Chaplin and Vittorio de Sica and Jean-Luc Goddard. We went to the Electric Cinema in Notting Hill Gate, a down-at-the-heels early movie palace that had a jerry-rigged ticket booth made out of plywood boards, painted pink. Atop the pink were green bubbles in which floated quotations from that font of all wisdom, Bob Dylan. From the Tube station at Notting Hill Gate it was a long trek to the Electric, and I pushed myself past the point of exhaustion to walk there. Why didn't I ever suggest that we catch a cab or a bus? I still thought walking was good for me, that it would make me stronger— even though I never got stronger. Years later I would read that only "thoroughbreds and old polios" will keep going until they drop. A couple of times I've done that, collapsed unto the ground with exhaustion, too worn out to take another step. I never fell down on our way to the Electric, but I came close. We went to West End cinemas, sitting in the cheap seats close to the front, craning our necks; we went to programs run by obscure film clubs. We went to film series run by the British Film Institute and local cinema societies. He lay with his head against my breast, and it seemed as if he was shrinking while I was growing, until I became a gigantic mother, as he shrank and curled against me. We spent more money than we had. Ben ran a shop he'd inherited from his parents, and there was always money in the till, he just reached his hand in and pulled it out. When we ate at the fancy steak place on Montserrat Road, the waiter addressed us as "sir" and "ma'am." If we were stoned when we went there, that would throw us into fits of giggles. We ate at the cheap working-class cafés—pronounced with defiant de-Frenchification as "caffs"—along the Lower Richmond Road, where the menus consisted of various combinations of bangers, bacon, beans, eggs, and toast. Ben didn't want there to be anything between us, not so much as a scrap of fabric, and if I slept in a T-shirt he'd beg me to take it off. I craved meat, but British meat always tasted strange to me, as if it had come from animals long past their prime. The hamburgers at the Wimpy Bars that dotted London were thin, steamed rather than grilled, and had a faintly metallic taste. I so longed for American food that when a Kentucky Fried Chicken opened in Camden Town I secretly took the Tube there and bought a breast with a side of cole slaw and mashed potatoes, and ate it out of the box on a park bench. And was, of course, disappointed. A hamburger place called the Great American Disaster opened on the Fulham Road in Chelsea, decorated with replicas of newspaper headlines telling of the sinking of the Titanic, the Hindenburg disaster, the stock market crash of '29, and serving not only ice water—just as was done in America—but hamburgers that tasted like the hamburgers I'd eaten at home. There was always a queue outside, and Ben and I would wait in it patiently, me leaning on my crutches, sometimes for hours. Sometimes I'd have a chocolate bar for breakfast and a packet of crisps—a bag of potato chips, in American—for lunch. I ate them mostly for the pleasure of at last being able to say, *This is my life, and I can do whatever I want.*

I never felt clean. It didn't matter how many baths I took, I felt gritty within minutes after stepping out of the tub. I bought a mauve maxidress and lace-up suede boots and had my hair cut in a shag. I was forever being asked, "Has anyone ever told you that you look like Jane Fonda?"

My mother sent me blue air letters, filled with news, weather reports, coming from an imaginary place we called home, as fake as one of the Potemkin villages, elaborate false villages built along the route of Catherine the Great's travels to convince her of the prosperity of her lands. Did my father ever write me a letter? I don't think so. He might have sent me a postcard, one of the three or four I have gotten from him in the course of my life, signed not "Love," but "Sincerely." It won't be until my father is seventy-nine years old that he will say the words "I love you" to me.

The front room of our flat was packed with bookshelves containing *Anna Karenina* and Timothy Leary's *The Politics of Ecstasy*. R. D. Laing's *Sanity, Madness and the Family. In the Fist of the Revolution,* a book extolling Castro's Cuba. We saw no contradiction in believing avidly in all sorts of revolutions—Leary's revolution via mind expansion, Laing's treatise on the need to overthrow the nuclear family, and the Cuban revolution. I can only imagine what might have happened to either Leary or the radical psychiatrist Laing had they found themselves in Castro's Cuba.

Also on the shelf was Nell Dunn's *Poor Cow*. Dunn was married to another writer, Jeremy Sandford, and Ben said he knew both of them. He didn't just know a *writer*, he knew *two* writers. Two writers who had actually *published* books. We dropped by their place one time, but no one seemed to be home, although we went around knocking on various doors and windows. I half hoped we'd go back there sometime, imagined Jeremy Sandford clapping Ben on the back, calling up the stairs, "Nell, come on down. Guess who's here?" But I half dreaded it, too, afraid one or the other of them might give him a quizzical look, not quite placing him, and when Ben reminded him of his name, their connection, then would give him a too-enthusiastic handshake, saying, "Oh, yes, yes! Great to see you! Unfortunately, we're just—just on our way out."

One night we were hitching home from the cinema—we must have got out so late that the Tube had stopped running—and caught a lift with a man driving a Jaguar, who asked where we were headed.

"Oh, Putney. I hear that's a pretty nice part of town."

"There's one grotty part," Ben said defensively. "That's where we live."

Along with our other political friends, I dutifully engaged in ritualized grumbling about trendies who owned cars, dressed in clothing they bought on the King's Road, decorating their houses with Japanese paper lampshades they bought at Habitat and drinking wine from matching glasses, assuaging their guilt by giving to Shelter or the Campaign for Nuclear Disarmament. We drank wine occasionally, but not only did we never have matching wineglasses—we drank out of the odds and ends of water glasses we'd accumulated—but we also never had a corkscrew, so opening the bottles always involved trying to wrench the cork out with nails or push it all the way into the bottle with a knife. Those trendies had well-appointed kitchens with teak cabinets and drawers they pulled open that contained not just corkscrews but matching cutlery.

We didn't look down on people who had picked up objects that were fanciful and beautiful in the markets of Marrakech or who could proclaim, when complimented on a sofa or antique table, "Ten quid at the Sally Army!" In this spirit, I determined to brighten up our surroundings by making a batik bedspread, having gotten the instructions from a book I checked out of the library, which described it as "An Easy Weekend Project!" The process involved melting blocks of paraffin—"CAREFUL," the instructions had warned, "overheating the wax may cause it to emit toxic smoke or burst into flames," which was one disaster I did manage to avoid. I then applied the melted wax to the areas of the muslin cloth I didn't want dyed, dunked the cotton in an enormous vat of dye and water heated on the stove, which I stirred away at with a wooden stick. The resemblance to the witches Macbeth encountered on the moor was not lost on me. The wet and waxy cloth had absorbed enough water that it was now heavy, and flopped like the body of a sea lion when I tipped the cauldron into the kitchen sink. "Rinse until the water runs clear," the directions advised, and I spent hours standing over the sink, running the water, squeezing and folding and wrestling with the fabric, my legs aching from standing for so long. Although the water never did run completely clear, I ventured on to the next step, and having squeezed out the excess water, hung the bedspread-to-be over the shower curtain rod in the bathroom. Did I get Ben to help me with this part of the project? I don't think I did. I must have dragged a wooden chair into the bathroom, and clambered up onto it. Reddish water trickled from it, splattering the tub, the linoleum floor.

How long did it hang there, drying but never quite getting dry, in that damp London flat? Several weeks, I think. Every now and again I'd feel the fabric, and it would still be damp. After a while I stopped even noticing it hanging there.

We dropped acid during a power blackout, our flat lit with candles. When Ben went into the bathroom, his hallucinations turned the bedspread into the skin of our cat, which he thought I had killed and skinned. On another acid trip, when I handed him a cup of tea, he thought I was handing him a cup of blood. But although I might be transformed into some mythological figure—a Kali, a Medea, a bloody-toothed mother who devoured her own children—in his LSD-fueled hallucinations, in the hard light of day he loved me. He loved me so much he could not live without me, loved me so much that he would die if I ever left him.

My second English winter set in. London is on the same latitude as New-foundland and Labrador, and as October seeped into November, November into December, the sun came up later and later, until, with the winter solstice drawing close, daybreak came at around ten in the morning, and dusk settled in before two in the afternoon. At the midmorning dawn, the color of the sky changed from slate to lead, while at dusk the leaden sky took on a cinereal cast. After long weeks without sight of the sun, while I never ceased to believe in its existence, it came to seem like the sort of cosmic phenomenon which one accepts the existence of without direct evidence, like the rings of Saturn and black holes.

Oh, the gloom of that winter! Oh, the sight of the corner greengrocers, where the scant winter vegetables were displayed—brussels sprouts and cabbage, along with miscellaneous root vegetables. Potatoes and carrots I knew from home, but there were also a variety of strange tubers in shades of chalk white, brown, and sulfur yellow, along with some warty gourds. They had medieval-sounding names—Jerusalem artichokes, swede, parsnips; I was never sure which word went with which vegetable. Many of the root vegetables had thin hair roots, making me think of the chins of wizened old men with a few long whiskers protruding.

Dripping—the grease from frying bacon, or culled from the bottom of a roasting pan—was not discarded but hoarded, and a common English supper was white bread spread with dripping, or white bread with margarine and sugar.

As the winter deepened, the faint sulfurous odor given off by the cabbages and brussels sprouts grew less and less faint. In the flats above and around us, our neighbors boiled those cruciferous vegetables, boiled them and boiled them and boiled them, and that smell seeped into our flat through the gap between the windowsill and the window proper, wafted under our door, settled around us like a low-hanging gas. I could not get rid of the foul taste in the back of my throat.

The English did not feel deprived by the scantiness of their food, by its plainness. They seemed to approach eating with the proud stoicism with which they approached so much else. George Orwell had summed up this attitude when he wrote, "A human being is primarily a bag for putting food into." To want spices in one's food, to yearn for central heating, to expect to reach the age of twenty-five without at least a mild case of lumbago or rheumatism, was to reveal oneself to be spoiled, coddled, American. It was this quality of self-denial that had enabled them to survive the horrors of the Blitz, the years of rationing that followed the end of WWII, this old don't-moan-and-carry-on-about-miseries-just-get-on-with-it attitude.

One day in the middle of that bleak winter—perhaps fueled by the speed we occasionally dropped—I tugged that batik bedspread down from the rod in the bathroom and undertook the next step of the process— removing the wax, which was to be done by spreading newspaper over the cloth and pressing it with an iron. The wax would melt and soak into the newspaper. The directions made it sound as if this was a process done once, but I spent hours and hours, spreading sheet after sheet of *The Guardian* on the bedspread, pressing down on the iron, getting that sheet of newsprint saturated with wax, laying down another sheet of newspaper, pressing down with the iron. Once I brought the iron down on my left hand by mistake, which left me with a triangle-shaped scar that lasted for years. As I inhaled the endless cigarettes I smoked, I also drew into my lungs the oily smell of hot wax.

Finally, at about three or four in the morning, I decided to call it quits. I gathered up the waxy newspapers from the floor, but when I crumpled them up to throw them away, they unleashed a shower of wax flakes, falling like snow on the gray wall-to-wall carpeting. The bedspread itself was still thick with wax, and I left it in a heap on the floor.

On the fourth or fifth day without so much as a glimpse of the sun, in October or maybe November, I had an afternoon-long attack of the blues.

That blue afternoon was followed by another one, a few days later, and before long a blue day stretched into a blue week that stretched into a blue month. My doctor diagnosed me, gave it a name—I was now officially Depressed. She wrote a prescription for me for antidepressants and arranged for me to see a psychiatrist, although there would be a six-week wait before I could get an appointment.

A stranger passing me on the street said, "Cheer up, love. It can't be as bad as all that."

Sometimes when I was riding the bus down Oxford Street or Fulham Road, the bus would stop at a red light, and I would have a minute or two to gaze into one of the shopwindows we were passing. I didn't yearn for the rooms filled with lace tablecloths, porcelain, and leaded crystal; but sometimes I'd stare into the scene of a wooden table, with place mats made of bamboo or rush, glazed earthenware plates, brightly colored Le Creuset pots and pans. In the center of the table there might be a basket from Bali or Nigeria. I glimpsed a world it seemed I could never enter—a world where nothing was chipped or cracked and nothing was cobbled together. The plates matched, the place mats matched. I pictured the life of the imaginary woman who had set that table—who seemed to be waiting, just beyond the back of the window display, who was about to enter—perhaps cradling an enormous wooden salad bowl, laughing at a joke she had just been told or calling over her shoulder to the perfect, nonexistent husband who was also waiting in the wings. She might be saying, "Oh, bugger, was that the doorbell? Don't tell me they're here already." That was the kind of thing the woman who lived in that shopwindow got upset about—guests arriving too early, the broccoli cooking a tad too long. She did not wonder how she could possibly survive another week of winter. She didn't feel perpetually unclean, always fighting against the chaos that engulfed her, although the harder she fought the more chaotic things became. The woman who lived this imaginary life did not have a husband who threatened to kill himself if she left him.

In the midst of that bleak, bleak winter, we went for a weekend visit to friends of Ben who lived in a thatched-roof cottage. I looked forward to the visit with a kind of desperate determination. We would get out of London, my foul mood would break as the weather sometimes broke, low-lying clouds being blown away by an unseen wind.

But when we stepped inside the cottage, the ceiling was just a few inches above my head.

As we exchanged pleasantries, I heard an odd pinging noise from above.

"Don't mind that, it's just the squirrels dropping acorns," our hostess said.

I was probably in the midst of answering the question "How big an island is Rhode Island?" when I heard an even stranger scritching sound.

"Damn rats."

Thatch roofing was as vexing as it was charming. All manner of vermin—especially rats—found it ideal for nesting. Old Harry—who I gathered was some kind of neighborhood handyman-and-tinker-cum-rat-killer—would be called soon to "make a good job of them."

We ate a Sunday joint, a piece of tough beef that had been cooked for hours, brussels sprouts that had been boiled with ferocity. I sawed away at the gray meat, then chewed away at it. The brussels sprouts had been cooked for so long they could have been gummed by the toothless. At the end of the meal I heard the words I'd come to dread: "Since you're American, I made coffee especially for you." We were then served coffee doctored with bitter chicory, along with milk that had been heated on the stove until it had undergone a good hearty boil. As it cooled, a skin formed on top of it, which was stirred back into the milk. I couldn't bear to drink the coffee without milk—and lots of sugar—but, just as I had feared, as I was gulping it down, a thin snake of milk, the remains of the skin, slithered down my throat.

We slept that night in a featherbed, an item of furniture I knew well from fairy tales. I had imagined something ethereal, verging on cloudlike. Instead, when we climbed into the enormous, feather-filled mattress, it rose up around us, enfolding us within it, pressing Ben's body against mine, a soft prison.

I look back on that Anne of nineteen and twenty from the lofty vantage point of all the decades that have passed, all that I have come to understand in those years. It is almost as if I have lifted the roof off that brick building on Lacy Road, as if it were some grotesque dollhouse, and peer down onto those miniature figures, "Anne" and "Ben." Time has given me such a vantage point that it feels right to talk about myself in the third person, a self so different she might as well be another. I can lay out, with near-mathematical precision, what was going wrong in the psyche of that troubled young woman.

On the most basic level, a tendency to depression that certainly has a biological component, exacerbated by seasonal affective disorder. Sometimes now I joke, "I have a remarkably simple emotional makeup. When the sun comes out from behind a cloud I'm happy, and when it goes back behind a cloud, I'm sad."

But those tendencies on their own were not enough to cause the collapse I was skirting the edges of. I had found myself a man—surprise, surprise!—who was an image of my father. A man who needed me, who loved me, who couldn't live without me, who loved me to death. And inside? My psyche was as fragile as a raw egg. It had been so important to my family that I come through the ordeal of polio unwounded, capable, competent, independent, that everything within me that was wounded, that was frail, that was needy was walled off. Add to that psychological stew the aftereffects of my father's violence.

But perhaps, having allowed the Anne-of-fifty-three to cast her cool eye on the Anne-of-twenty, I should allow the tables to be turned. What would that Anne think of this one?

Did I imagine myself at fifty-three? I think forty seemed the edge of the earth, the boundary of imagination. At twenty I pictured myself living in a Victorian house with too many rooms, like the house where we lived in Providence, the houses where I babysat. But unlike my parents' house, this Victorian wouldn't be overstuffed and dark. It would be filled with light and spareness. My table would be set with thick, handmade pottery dishes and the walls decorated with handwoven baskets from Bali or Nepal. And although I said I never wanted children, and never imagined myself pregnant, and above all never undergoing that gross, sowlike act of giving birth, in those fantasies there were always five or six vague children, off in the distance. And, of course, a husband. Equally vague, but certainly not the man I was married to then.

What would that Anne have made of my aloneness, of my single child, of the cool modern space I occupy, so far removed from the big ramshackle house I once imagined?

But before that Anne noticed any of that, her eyes would be riveted by the bright red wheelchair in which I sit. Anne-of-twenty, it was all a lie—all that hard work and pushing yourself to the point of exhaustion won't make you better—in fact, you are doing just the opposite, wearing out your fragile muscles every time you force yourself to hike the exhausting distance between the Notting Hill Gate Tube station and the Electric Cinema, every time you tell yourself, "Just swim one more lap, one more."

But the wheelchair I sit in now was literally unimaginable. After all, in fantasies of the future medicine cured us; we didn't get cool new equipment, in flashy colors and with engineering derived from, of all things, hang gliders. In the hospital the wheelchairs were made of wicker and wood. Even the guys who came back from Vietnam as paras and quads were riding clunky chairs. It wouldn't be until 1978, when Marilyn Hamilton became paralyzed in a hang-gliding accident and was given one of these clunkers that the industry was revolutionized. Nor can that Anne of so many years ago imagine that there will be curb cuts, accessible bathrooms, that when she passes another disabled person on the street she will meet their gaze and greet them, that SDS will no longer stand for Students for a Democratic Society but Society for Disability Studies, that at their annual conference she will dance in her wheelchair with other twisting, flailing, wild disabled bodies.

No, Anne-of-twenty can't imagine that future. She can't imagine much of a future at all. She just knows she wants to get away.

Some mornings I would wake up and lie in bed and think: If he started hating me, I could get away. What would I have to do to get him to hate me? I could stop washing. I could stuff myself full of food. I could stop speaking to him. I could lie still and lifeless under him while he had sex with me. If I did those things, would he start hating me and let me go?

HUMPTY-DUMPTY

I didn't do any of those things. I just got more and more depressed. Depressed enough that I got admitted to a psych hospital.

So, at nineteen, I spent a second six months in a hospital, just as I had when I was three. Both the name of the hospital, Atkinson Morley's, and its address, Copse Hill in Wimbledon, had a quaint Victorian air. The hospital itself had been built in the middle of the nineteenth century, but it was as utterly plain and devoid of excess ornament as a Bauhaus structure. Dickens had memorialized such drab Victorian architecture in *Hard Times*: "The jail might have been the infirmary, the infirmary might have been the jail, the town-hall might have been either, or both." For all the grimness of its facade, the hospital presented its best face to the street. The floors inside were covered with gray linoleum, and the double-paned windows, stretching almost from floor to ceiling, had what appeared to be chicken wire between the panes of glass, to make them unbreakable. A twenty-bed women's ward was on one side of the corridor and a twenty-bed men's ward on the other. An honest institution, at least, one that didn't pretend to be anything else.

On my first day there, one of the other patients—a beautiful long-haired woman wearing a Moroccan caftan—came up to me and comforted me as I cried, asking me what was wrong.

"I was remembering," I said, "my father choking me. When I was a kid. I thought he was going to kill me." Was it really the first time I had said those words aloud?

She put her arm around me. "Does it help you to know that you are here with us now? That you're safe now?"

My images of mental hospitals had been derived from the sight of Rhode Island's grim state institutions, a photographic exposé in *Look* magazine called "Christmas in Purgatory," and movies like *The Snake Pit,* of which I had seen a few scenes on the fuzzy screen of our black-and-white TV. The snake pit referred to an ancient method of treatment—lowering an insane person into a snake pit in an attempt to cure her or his insanity. I had taken it much more literally, forming an image of mental patients themselves lying on the floor, writhing in agony. Atkinson Morley's seemed more like a summer camp, an impression that was strengthened when I began to join the others my age, wandering down to the rugby pitch behind the hospital to smoke dope. Alert to the perils of institution-alization, the staff encouraged us to go into the village of Wimbledon, and I returned nearly every weekend to that grim flat.

My fellow patients were former actresses whose careers had hit the skids; a handful of schizophrenics; more than a few depressed young women, my age or a little bit older; an elderly woman with a title, suffer-ing from what was then called presenile dementia—what today would probably be diagnosed as early-onset Alzheimer's.

The hospital was a therapeutic community. The notion was that rather than therapy being limited to individual sessions with one's therapist, healing would take place on a twenty-four-hour-a-day basis—or at least sixteen hours, given that we had to sleep. Sometimes the nonstop therapy tilted over into the ridiculous. On one of my first days there, a nurse came over as I was making my bed, and said, "Let me give you a hand . . . I'm Mary. What's your name?"

I swallowed hard. When I was in a depression, my normal charm and volubility disappeared, and even speaking became hard for me. I would become afraid I was going to mispronounce a word, and my throat would tighten with anxiety.

"Anne," I managed to say, although my voice caught midway through the word.

"Ian?" she asked, puzzled.

There. It had happened. I couldn't even say my own name right. "Anne," I repeated, almost in a whisper. "A-n-n-e."

"Oh, sorry," she said briskly. "I guess it's your American accent. I thought you said 'Ian.'"

"So," she said, tucking the bottom of the sheet under the mattress. "What's your problem?"

"I'm—I'm depressed," I managed to mutter after a few minutes.

"That's your *symptom*," she said, as she smoothed the wrinkles out of the sheet. "What's *causing* your depression?" I had no idea. I felt as if I were taking a final exam and could not begin to answer the essay question that would count for the bulk of my grade. I began to shake with fear. What had happened to that other Anne, the one all the grown-ups thought was so mature, the one who got on a plane and flew off to Europe to live on her own at the age of eighteen? Did these two personalities really co-exist within the same sack of skin?

I longed to have some easily encapsulated "problem," as some of my ward mates did—a pathological maternal attachment, intractable grief following the loss of a partner. Trying to define what had gone wrong for me seemed as difficult as trying to find a geometrical term for the shape of a cloud. In reaction to Freudianism's focus on childhood and the uncovering of child roots for emotional ills, the therapeutic focus was on the here and now. My presenting problem, my here-and-now issue—although it took me months and months to articulate it fully—was my desire to get free of that marriage. The path that had led me to that disastrous marriage was barely explored.

It wasn't all wafting about in caftans, smoking dope on the rugby pitch, and endlessly yammering about our problems, though. Electroshock therapy was given to some of those who were depressed—not, thankfully, to me, as the cure seemed worse than the disease, with patients numb and disoriented afterward. A few patients with intractable anxiety found themselves given a more sophisticated version of a lobotomy in the neurosurgical unit downstairs.

Atkinson Morley's was my asylum, in the best sense of the word. It was there that I began to get the strength to leave that disastrous marriage. My resolve never lasted for long—Ben would start threatening suicide, and I'd feel guilty and go back to him.

Was my depression genetic? Almost certainly it was, at least in some measure. Depression must have been part of my father's emotional distress, and his alcoholism may in part have been a result of using gin and whiskey to get some relief from his raging sorrow. And all but one of my siblings has struggled with depression—although what that proves is far from definitive, given that all of my siblings shared an upbringing that was a near-perfect recipe for inducing depression.

How much was due to the polio itself, for polio is a disease not just of the motor neurons but of the brain, although this is an aspect of the virus that was largely suppressed in the creation of the social myths of polio. A 1990 survey of polio survivors revealed that a quarter of them had been diagnosed with clinical depression. But while that raises the possibility of a direct link between polio itself and depression, nearly all people who had polio experienced traumatic separations from their families, along with the wounds—both physical and emotional—of subsequent surgeries, and the ongoing injury of finding themselves in severely constrained social roles. In addition the pressure on people who'd had polio to minimize the extent of their disability, to be cheerful overcomers, to fit themselves into the normal world, often resulted in a bifurcated self. Alongside the self who was competent, precociously mature, and strong, another, more shadowed self lived—sensitive to criticism, fearful of being unable to live up to the world's expectations, and above all, lonely, for this was the part of ourselves we were supposed to keep well hidden. Another near-perfect recipe for creating emotional distress.

What were the effects of polio on the brain? Bulbar polio—polio that manifested primarily in the bulb-shaped stem of the brain—was the most dangerous sort of polio, for "bulbars"—as they were sometimes called by hospital staff—could lose their ability to swallow and even to breathe. Bulbar polio was seen as a distinct form of the disease, although in fact nearly everyone who had a clinical case of polio had brain involvement. Dr. David Bodian, a prominent polio researcher, wrote more than half a century ago: "All available evidence shows conclusively that every case of polio exhibits damage in the brain." What polio affected was not cognitive functioning, but the brain stem, which, in addition to regulating breathing and swallowing, also controls such higher-level functions as alertness and the sleep/wake cycle, as well as blood pressure, heart rate, and muscle tone. Most of us who had had polio didn't know anything about brain involvement until we began to hear about it, decades after our initial experience with the disease, as a possible cause of postpolio fatigue.

To understand why polio's effects on the brain were so long ignored, we need to look not only to how the narrative about polio was formed, but how the narrative of disease itself changed as the nineteenth century gave way to the twentieth. Read any nineteenth-century novel, and a view of disease very different from our own comes into focus. Disease was not seen primarily through the lens of medicine but had a weight that was moral, spiritual. The person with a disease was not going through a medical crisis but a crisis of the soul. Koch's revolution—sharply defining disease, seeing it as caused by a specific microbe—meant also a narrowing of the effects of disease on the body. Disease was no longer diffused throughout the self but limited to specific bodily processes.

This shift is illustrated in Alan Marshall's *I Can Jump Puddles*, an account of Marshall's history with polio in the early 1900s in Australia. His neighbors "associated the word 'Paralysis' with idiocy, and the query, 'Have you heard if his mind is affected?' was asked from many a halted buggy."

One of the steps in the creation of polio as the disease that could be overcome with hard work, hard work, and more hard work, the disease whose survivors were usually accepted back into their communities and families—was to define it as a disease whose effects were limited to the obvious and the physical. We were not "crippled inside" but only outside. The cores of us, the essence of who we were, were to remain the nondisabled selves we had been prior to polio. To suggest how deeply the disease itself had affected us—etching whorls into our brains, or to look at the enormous psychological damage caused by medical procedures, was to threaten that. Eleanor Roosevelt, asked if polio had affected her husband's mind, gave an exemplary answer: "How could it be otherwise? One couldn't suffer as my husband has suffered and failed to be affected. Suffering has made him more sensitive, more responsive to his fellow men."

And, after all, the associations raised by the phrase "brain damage" are frightening ones. Say the words "brain damage" and what do you picture? Back wards of institutions? Lenny in *Of Mice and Men*? An unkempt figure, stuttering and lurching? Blank stupidity? We didn't seem, in any superficial ways, to be exhibiting any such signs of brain damage. Sometimes it even seemed that polio made kids smarter. Children who had paid scant attention to schoolwork, imagining futures as firemen, blue-collar workers, nurses, mothers, began to study hard, knowing that their minds, not their physical prowess, would be what they would rely on as adults.

Finally I left the hospital and left England—flying home on a sixty-eight-dollar charter flight between London and New York. The plan was that Ben would later follow me, when he'd sold a piece of property he owned. I called my parents from New York to tell them I'd arrived, and had booked a flight on a relatively new commuter airline from there to Providence. "It's on Pilgrim, and it gets in—" I said to my father.

"Pilgrim? There's no Pilgrim Airline. What does it say on your ticket jacket?"

"Pilgrim," I said.

"No, no," he said. "Go back to the ticket counter. Ask them what the real name is."

I stood in the phone booth, holding the solid black receiver in my hand, on the verge of tears. He must have been drunk, I now realize. Once he had said, "Pilgrim? There's no Pilgrim Airline," his pride wouldn't allow him to back down. When I insisted he was wrong, he—emperor of his crazy, fragile kingdom—could see my assertion only as an attack. I clutched the phone, wondering how I could go back to the ticket counter, with the sign above it that read "Pilgrim," and ask them what their real name was, because my father didn't believe me? Would someone be there at the airport to meet me when my plane landed in Providence?

Somehow I got my sister Sandra on the phone, gave her the time my flight arrived.

Within two weeks I was lying in a coma, my life in danger, having swallowed an overdose of antidepressants.

I had gone to the psychiatrist my father had seen "when he was quitting smoking," as my mother put it, using her euphemism for the time of our lives when he had been floridly mentally ill.

The doctor had been in the middle of writing me a prescription for antidepressants—one of the old-fashioned tricyclics that preceded today's Prozac and Zoloft, which were far more dangerous if one took a deliberate overdose—and asked me, "You've never tried to hurt yourself, have you?"

"Not really," I said. "Well—when I was in junior high school, I used to swallow handfuls of aspirin and cut my wrists with a razor blade. It's funny—I've never told anybody that before." Not only was I telegraphing him a distress signal, but it is well known that the period after being discharged from the safe haven of a psych hospital is a time when anyone is particularly vulnerable to suicide, especially an adolescent.

When I came to several days after taking the overdose, the groggy, underwater feeling was familiar, as was the setting. "Is my operation over?" I asked the nurse.

"You didn't have an operation," she said. "Do you remember what happened?"

I remembered being in my friend's apartment, swallowing the yellow pills. And then I tumbled back down into a groggy semicoma. I learned later that I had almost died the night of the overdose.

When I woke up again, my mother was sitting next to my bed, just as she had so many times before when I broke the surface from the deep waters of a stuporous sleep. And then I remembered what had happened and felt overwhelmed with guilt, knowing the pain I had caused my family.

After my suicide attempt, my mother told me often that she loved me. These were words I had never heard from her before—although I had always known that she loved me. And then she would say, "You can't leave Ben. He loves you so much." She also told me several times, "I don't feel guilty that you tried to kill yourself." She sounded almost defiant when she said this. How can your child come close to dying in a suicide attempt and you feel no guilt? Maybe my mother felt so overwhelmed by guilt she couldn't begin to feel a fraction of it? Or maybe if she knew her own guilt, she'd have to experience my father's guilt, too? It remains one of those mysterious responses from her that I still can't figure out.

My mother loves my son and felt the gap in her life when we were all in our thirties and she had no grandchildren. But when I called to tell her I was pregnant, that she would at last have a grandchild, she said, "Oh." I waited in the silence for her say something more, and finally she did. "What have you been doing politically?" I wondered if perhaps one of my sisters, who had struggled with infertility, was in the same room when she got the call. But if that was the case, then why didn't she call me back later and tell me that? Was it something to do with my disability? Of course I could have said, "What's going on? Why aren't you happy for me?" I suppose I didn't because I know her well enough that I know she'd reply, in a flat voice, "Oh, I'm happy." And if I had said, "You don't sound very happy," I would have come smack up against her denial.

After my overdose my mother arranged for me to see another doctor. This one turned out to be downright bizarre. Once, for instance, he interrupted me in midsentence, as I was talking about my fears about speaking in class—I was taking a film history class at Rhode Island College—with: "Hey. Do you want to know how to remember the difference between stalactites and stalagmites? Stalagmites hang down from the ceiling of a cave, and the *g* in stalagmites hangs down." That he had it backward— stalagmites form on the floors of caves—was the least of it. He also answered his phone whenever it rang—this despite having a secretary in the next room—so often most of our sessions would be given over to me sitting there while he counseled someone else on the telephone, or scheduled appointments. Hanging up the phone, he might turn to me and say, indicating the telephone, about the person he had just been conversing with, "What a narcissistic bitch! Maybe you know her," and he'd proceed to tell me her name. Or he might say, "Now this patient's really interesting. Got a phobia about fish. Fish, of all things."

For a few months I didn't do much besides watch television and eat and visit my nutty psychiatrist. Sit-com reruns. The *Dick Cavett Show*. Old movies. Wise potato chips dipped in sour cream, Cheetos, Reese's peanut butter cups. I didn't brush my hair. I wanted to be ugly and never, ever have to be loved again. Ben kept sending me letters, but I didn't answer them. After a while I stopped opening them. One day he called—a transatlantic phone call was a big deal in those days—and I had my brother tell him I wasn't home.

My father knew that I wanted to be a writer, and over and over he asked me, "So when are you going to get something published?" It was his way of expressing interest, but to me it had sounded like a taunt. It was a question I could only answer with an "I don't know." A few times he asked me this question when we were driving in the car, and the image flashed across my mind of me pulling open the car door, and throwing myself onto the highway.

I moved out of my parents' house and in with a friend. Every morning the alarm would wake me in my rumpled bed. The bottom sheet had long since come untucked, and so I lay half on it wrinkled beneath me, half on the bare mattress. I would vow that *this* day, when I got home from work, I would not only make the bed, I would pick up the coffee cups that had been left with an inch or so of coffee in the bottom, left for weeks until they were dotted with colonies of blue-green mold. It wouldn't take that long to get my room cleaned up—not if I really applied myself. I'd get the bed made and the coffee cups washed out, the dirty clothes picked up from the floor and stuffed into a pillowcase to take over to my mother's.

And then the knowledge that yesterday morning I had made those same resolutions, and the morning before that, and the morning before that, and the morning before that would wash over me. I had failed a hundred times before at these tasks that were seemingly simple tasks.

I took menial jobs. For a day and a half I even worked as a telephone solicitor selling lightbulbs, which were supposed to last five years and were sold by "the handicapped." Although the set speech we were given to read said, "We are not looking for a handout . . . ," that was manifestly what we were doing. Even now, thirty years later, a sense of shame washes over me as I write about this: Even now, with my advanced degrees and the books I have published and the awards I have won, I feel the pain of having been reduced to doing that, so sharp I have to fight to keep myself from going to wash the dishes, vacuum the floor, clean out my closets— anything but write about this.

When I applied for the job I lumbered up the stairs on my crutches and entered the room—with rows of school desks with a black telephone on each one. The man who was in charge grinned when he saw me. It was the opposite of the reaction I was used to from men in suits who hire and fire workers. Nearly all the other people who were making these phone calls had psychiatric impairments, including one woman who was so dopey with antipsychotic medications that she kept falling asleep in mid-sentence. I was the sort of handicapped person the people on the other end of the phone pictured. For hours and hours on end, I dialed phone numbers, reading off my prepared spiel from the mimeographed sheet in front of me. I didn't return from my break midway through my second evening.

I worked factory jobs, easy to get in Rhode Island in those days. I had figured out that if I walked into a personnel office without my crutches, I crossed a line from the world of the handicapped to the world of the normal. I loaded Bic pens into cartons in a factory, standing on my feet for eight hours a day. It would have been perfectly easy for me to do the job perched on a stool, but I didn't dare to ask for one, afraid I'd be fired if I did so. The cards onto which the Bic pens were laminated covered my fingers with paper cuts, and I remember the feel of those cuts on my fingers, the sight of my fingertips, wrapped with Band-Aids. I don't remember what my legs felt like after standing on them for eight hours a day, but I know they must have ached and ached. The lower half of my body was terra incognita, a land without words. To have spoken of my aching legs would have been to break that compact I—along with so many others who had had polio—had made with the world—not to complain, to be a good sport, to soldier on, not to whine, to just keep going.

My housemate, Maggie, and I got jobs together at a jewelry factory. Factories in Rhode Island in those days always had signs out in front that said NOW HIRING! STRINGERS, CARDERS, WRAPPERS, FOOT PRESS OPERATORS. The woman in personnel tried to talk us into working the foot press, but Maggie was adamant. Being a foot-press operator paid better, but few foot-press operators retired from their jobs with all their fingers intact— getting at least one lopped off in a machine was almost inevitable. Once, at a reading in California, I read a short story set in Rhode Island, and the reader who followed me said, "I'm from Rhode Island, too," and held up his hand to show me his missing digits, displaying our state symbol. Instead we worked as carders, which meant we took the cheap costume jewelry—which was wheeled into our department in the kinds of cloth bins that institutions move laundry around in. It was piecework, meaning if you got fast enough at it, you could make more than the minimum wage, although neither of us ever managed to do that. Nixon had just made his trip to China, the first U.S. president to do so since the Communist regime had been established in 1949, and so that summer there were various items of jewelry that referenced China—bracelets with black-and-white pandas dangling from them, earrings in the shape of bamboo and Chinese calligraphy, along with the less topical lucky-penny ponytail holders and fake gold hoop earrings that sold at Woolworth's for $1.29. At least here we could talk or listen to the radio, which made the time pass. In other parts of the factory—and when I worked packing Bic pens—the machinery was so loud that conversation was impossible.

I moved to Boston, started taking classes at Harvard Extension, working—sometimes as a cabdriver, sometimes as a temporary office worker. I got divorced. At times it seemed I was putting my life back together; at other times my hold was tenuous indeed. I was aware of people whom mental illness and/or some other cataclysm had cast adrift from the safe harbor of middle-class life, and who spent decades drifting, working menial jobs, never able to return to the solid life that had seemed their birthright. Would I end up like that? Perhaps I wasn't a writer doing a temporary stint as a file clerk but a file clerk with illusions of being a writer.

The lessons I had learned from polio rehabilitation here stood me in good stead. Work hard. Keep trying. Don't give up. Never say die. I engaged in psychotherapy with the same kind of desperate hope with which I had once embarked on physical therapy.

When I saw another disabled person I still crossed the street, or at least set my pace so that no passerby would think that we were together, two cripples out on a day pass from some institution, two members of some pathetic club for rejects. I got angry at other disabled people I saw on the street with their clunking, awkward crutches and braces. They always looked ugly to me. In truth, I think in those days, the early 1970s, most of us were still following the advice we'd been given about avoiding loud prints and clothing that drew attention to itself, so we were dressing like dowagers when we were in our twenties.

Was I even vaguely aware of the burgeoning disability-rights movement? I don't think so. It seemed natural to me, in those days before accessible parking, that I would have to leave myself an extra hour or so before my night classes at Harvard. Half an hour to find a parking place close enough that I could manage the walk, and then half an hour to walk my slow, slow walk from the car to my class.

I was so scared of men that sometimes when I was in a romantic situation I started to shake uncontrollably. I hardly had any clothes, mostly what I'd pulled out of the wooden box set out on the corner of Somerville Avenue and Prospect Street with the word FREE stenciled on it in black letters. I put together enough classes to get a bachelor's degree, and applied to graduate programs in creative writing. Every grad school application I filled out asked about "physical handicap," as it was put in those days.

Some of them added the phrase, "that would affect your education," and in that case I could honestly answer the question "No." But if that qualifying phrase wasn't added, I mentioned the polio, doing all I could to minimize it. Every school that knew about my disability rejected me, and, with one exception, every one that didn't accepted me. I was offered a fellowship from Stanford, and in August of 1976, my sister Jane and I set off for the West Coast—she had just graduated from college and was on her way to Seattle to join her girlfriend, Carla.

I had joined Triple A and had a Trip Tik made for me, a spiral-bound book one flipped through as one went along one's journey—a bit of over-preparation, since basically one got on I-80 and stayed on it from outside Altoona, Pennsylvania, to San Francisco. Having the Trip Tik made me feel very adult, as did the phrase "graduate student," although my anxiety about my future had coalesced into a fear of bridges and the downgrades of mountain highways. As we crept across Kansas and Nebraska, I kept imagining a long straight highway shooting down from the Sierras, at the bottom of which there would be a stoplight. I would brake the car furiously, hitting the brake with all my might, and still the car wouldn't even slow, and I would hurtle through the red light. I never pictured the aftermath—just the moment of sheer panic as I was unable to stop the car. We ate at Burger King and McDonald's, because those were the cheapest places to eat, and stayed at Motel 6s or other cheap motels with thin bars of soap and even thinner towels.

In 1973 Congress had passed a Rehabilitation Act that included a section—Section 504—outlawing discrimination against people with disabilities in any program receiving federal funds. Four years later the regulations setting forth what constituted discrimination had still not been signed. If a city ran a bus without a wheelchair lift, was that discrimination? Were universities required to hire readers to read textbooks to blind students? Activists were pushing, without any success, for the "enabling regs," as they were called, to be signed.

During my second semester at Stanford, in April 1976, disabled activists held demonstrations across the country, demanding that 504 be implemented. Sit-ins were held in Washington, D.C., New York, L.A., and San Francisco. In every other city the sit-ins ended at the end of the day, but at the Department of Health, Education, and Welfare in San Francisco, demonstrators decided not to leave—to make their protest more than symbolic. Headlines about the demonstration were on the front page of the *San Francisco Chronicle,* and I used to think, with that intemperance to which I was so prone, "I should drop out of school and go and join the sit-in." At the same time I was scared to even drive up to the city—less than an hour away—and join a support picket line. I wasn't sure I was disabled enough to really count. I was convinced that those disabled demonstrators, in their wheelchairs, carrying their white canes, were radically different from me.

While people who took part in the nearly monthlong sit-in had a variety of impairments, the early disability-rights movement was dominated by people who were polio survivors, like Ed Roberts and Judy Heumann. We shared a common experience of having been told that hard work would enable us to return to the world of the "normal." We had heard over and over again about one of us having been president. We were raised in the belief that we could do anything we set our minds to. Great things were expected of us. We then found our way blocked by a myriad of legal obstacles. Ed Roberts had initially been denied assistance from the California Department of Vocational Rehabilitation, which deemed him "too severely disabled" ever to work. A decade and a half after that, Roberts became head of the agency that had once said he was too disabled to hold a job. In 1970 Judy Heumann had been forced to file suit in federal court because she had been denied a New York teacher's license on account of her disability. Judy—who had gone on to become a Senate employee—had also been arrested in 1975 for boarding an airplane without either a nondisabled companion or a doctor's note certifying that she was able to fly unaccompanied. Nearly all public buildings were inaccessible to users in wheelchairs or to anyone who couldn't climb stairs.

Media attention reflected the spirit of the times. When Ed Roberts started at UC Berkeley—instead of staying in a dorm he slept in his iron lung at Cowell Health Center—the headline in a local paper described him as a "Helpless Cripple." The *New York Times*—which ran an editorial supporting Judy Heumann in her fight to get licensed as a teacher—nonetheless casually referred to her as a "polio victim."

As well as being born of the collision between high expectations and grim reality, the emerging movement for disability rights had been shaped by the social movements of the 1950s and 1960s—particularly the civil rights movement—with their examples of previously powerless sectors of society winning enormous changes by engaging in collective action. There were other, more direct connections with the civil rights movement, which we were not aware of at the time. For instance, the murder of fourteen-year-old Emmett Till in 1955 had been one of the galvanizing events of the civil rights movement. Although Till's short life became legendary, few knew that Till had been left with a speech impairment as a result of a bout with bulbar polio. His mother had taught him, when he had trouble speaking, to whistle in order to get his throat muscles to relax. Visiting relatives in Mississippi from his Chicago home, Till had been tortured and then murdered for having whistled at a white woman. His mother, Mamie Mobley, insisted on an open coffin for her son, wanting to make the brutality of Southern racism visible, and African American newspapers ran pictures on their front pages of his swollen and battered face. Until her death Mobley believed that the whistle leading to her son's death had been the result of an attempt to free his voice, rather than a wolf whistle directed at a white woman.

Another direct link between the disability movement and the black liberation movement was that the 504 sit-in would not have succeeded without the assistance of the Black Panthers, one of whose members was a participant. The Panthers were the ones who provided food to the demonstrators, undoing plans to starve the demonstrators out.

The women's movement, with its insistence that areas of life that had been seen as personal were in fact political, also struck chords within many of us. We looked inside as well as outside: Were the self-hatred and shame that so many of us experienced not a natural response to disability but a product of oppressive social relations?

While I was going to Stanford, I moved into a ramshackle wooden house—a somewhat funkier version of the house I'd imagined myself living in as a woman of forty, and fell in love—for the first time since my marriage had ended—with one of my housemates, a man named Mark. Mark was four years younger than I—still shy of twenty-one. I fell in love with him because he was gentle and quiet and always tentative about our relationship. He was a runner and didn't even smoke dope, because he worried smoking anything would affect his lungs. Here was a man who would never threaten to kill himself if I left him, who would never drop acid and think that I had killed the cat, skinned it, and draped its hide across the shower curtain.

His parents had been fundamentalist Christians who followed God's directive to be fruitful and multiply. They had nine kids—ten, if you counted their first baby, Lucille, who had died of pneumonia when she was six months old. Once, going through some old boxes of their papers in a garage in Seattle, we found a mimeographed newsletter put out by the Bible college they'd both attended, which included a letter from his mother. "The good Lord sent our sweet baby Lucille to live with us for six months, then took her home to live with Him forever in glory." In the Pentecostal churches, the Holy Spirit would descend on some of the worshippers, who would start speaking in tongues and writhing on the floor. Both hell and salvation itself seemed terrifying.

His parents had both been killed in an automobile accident when he was twelve. The accident had occurred on a family trip—the first time they had ever left the state of Washington. Mark and his younger brother had both broken their backs, and spent months in body casts in a hospital in Little Rock, Arkansas, alone, far from relatives.

I was drawn to his gentleness, to his sad, downcast eyes, in which you could see the hint of a Native American grandmother.

I wish there had been a moment when, like Saul on the road to Damascus, the scales fell from my eyes and I saw the truth in a blinding light. My journey toward the disability-rights movement had few dramatic moments.

After I finished the yearlong program at Stanford, Mark and I moved to San Francisco. At a meeting in San Francisco's City Hall, I struck up a conversation with a woman in a wheelchair. Because she couldn't write, she asked me to write down my name and phone number for her: "And write on the card that you're disabled," she said. I can only imagine the look of startled horror that must have passed over my face, because she muttered something: "Or that you have a handicap, or, uh . . ."

A while after that I went to see a charming French movie called *Diabolo Menthe*—*Peppermint Soda* was the English translation—about a thirteen-year-old French girl. The movie was warm and episodic, and the next morning, I got up and started jotting down my own memories from my thirteenth year, which coalesced into a short story I called "Like the

Hully-Gully But Not So Slow"—the title was taken from a line in a song I used to hear on the radio. I wrote about having an older sister who, like Sandra, seemed to know all the rules about being a teenager, and whom I regarded with both longing and contempt. I wrote about helping my Catholic friends with their catechism and how I'd longed to live in a world like theirs, where the question "Why are we on earth?" had a multipart answer that could be ticked off on one's fingers. I wrote about reading advertisements in the back of the *Times Magazine* for a sect called the Rosicrucians, which sometimes had the headline, "Your Thoughts Have Wings." A line drawing showed a man with a look of studious concentration and winged orbs flying out from his forehead, and the copy underneath explained how you could beam your thoughts into the minds of others. Sometimes at the dinner table, when my father would go into a rage over Sandra's friends calling during dinnertime, I'd start trying to beam my thoughts across the East Side. "Don't call Sandra Finger. Don't call her. Don't call Sandra Finger."

And I didn't make the central character nondisabled. I left her in braces and on crutches, and had the fictional older sister yell at her, as Sandra had once yelled at me, "Would you goddamn oil yourself? You were coming down the hall today, and everybody could hear you squeaking." It wasn't the first story I'd written in which disability appeared. But as an undergraduate I'd gotten the not-so-subtle message that this was a subject to be avoided. My professors told me that such stories were sentimental or that I was unfairly trying to win sympathy for my character by making her handicapped. In fairness to my professors those first attempts at writing about disability may well have been sentimental—after all, in the literary models I had in which disabled characters appeared, we were either read as grotesque, wounded, bitter—Captain Ahab being the ur-example—or sweet and sentimental—like Tiny Tim. I wish I had those early attempts so I could look at them from the vantage point provided by time, but I was so ashamed of them that I threw them out.

A little while before I wrote the story that proved to be a turning point for me, I'd joined a women writers' group that had originally formed within the creative writing program at San Francisco State in the early 1970s. They'd come together to protest the fact that, while students were required to write a paper on a major poet, not a single woman poet—not even Emily Dickinson—was considered major. Mostly when I look back on my days in the Women Writers Union, I cringe when I think of our self-righteousness, our self-importance, how our political outlook would lead us to praise some truly awful—but politically right-on—work. Once, I told Tede—my friend who would later die of AIDS—to introduce me at a reading as "a clerical worker and a cultural worker," which I meant ironically and thought would get a laugh, only to see the audience nod their heads solemnly. But it was in the Women Writers Union that I really found my voice as a disabled writer.

And finally, after years of avoiding other disabled people, I actually started making friends with other people with disabilities. When I was in my early thirties, reports about increasing fatigue and weakness in people who had had polio were just beginning to surface—the collection of symptoms now known as postpolio syndrome—I went to a conference for people who'd had polio. I felt like an adoptee meeting her birth family for the first time at an enormous family reunion. Here I was surrounded by people who shared my personality quirks—my tough sense of humor, my drive, my big smile, my anger.

PPS

Back when I was a child, even into my adulthood, at the end of letters there was sometimes the abbreviation "P.S." And occasionally, after that, a "P.P.S."—"postpostscript," my mother explained. PPS. It always made me giggle—partly because it contained the slightly naughty word "pee-pee," partly because it sounded simultaneously Latinate and silly. Now, of course, when nearly all letters are processed through a computer, after-thoughts are blended flawlessly into the text.

Now PPS means "postpolio syndrome."

My doctor handed me a prescription. Was it for physical therapy? Or an occupational therapy evaluation? I don't remember. What I do remember are the words in the upper-lefthand corner: Dx: PPS. I knew that "Dx" meant "diagnosis," and I knew that PPS meant "postpolio syndrome," but this was the first time I had seen that word officially applied to me. And even though I knew the answer to the question, still I asked her: "Does that mean 'postpolio syndrome'?"

"No," she said. "It stands for 'postpolio sequelae.' I don't really think the concept of postpolio syndrome is a useful one. I think it makes more sense to think of polio as a progressive neurological condition combined with chronic joint deterioration."

It's one of those moments of my life I remember with startling clarity, the way I remember the first time I said the words "my son," the way I remember my friend Barbara's body lying in her coffin, the memories calling back a whole train of associations: the taste of the cheddar-on-whole-wheat sandwich I was buying in the health food store when I said "my son" for the first time, the suddenness of the sob that racked me as I stood looking at Barb, the feeling of someone else's arms wrapping around me—I never knew whose—comforting me. I remember it that way, the sunny morning in San Francisco when I opened the door to see the manila envelope lying facedown on the doormat, and assumed it was a rejected manuscript; picked it up hoping for at least a letter rather than a simple printed slip, turned it over to see that it was a magazine I'd ordered, *Rehabilitation Gazette,* because it had an article about "premature aging" in people who'd had polio. Did this mean my hair was going to turn totally gray before I reached the age of forty? Would I have an old woman's lines on my face and jowls? Would my body, which had leaped so precipitously into womanhood leap just as precipitously out of it? I was twenty-nine that morning in Noe Valley, just saying good-bye to my youth and suddenly confronted with old age.

And that was the beginning of this second leg of the journey. No more was I the person of whom friends would say, "I don't think of you as handicapped," which, even though you understood it to be as politically offensive as "I don't think of you as gay," or "I don't think of you as a woman," still, secretly, pleased me. An identity held at an arm's length: I was no longer the one reaching out to embrace the identity of "disabled person"; now the disease was reaching out to embrace me.

I moved from the liminal space that straddled identities, my left foot in the world of the normals, my right foot in the world of cripples. My body, as well as my social identity, had been bifurcated: I had a good leg and a bad leg. Sometimes I personified those two sisters who were my lower limbs, my good girl and my bad girl, as Sonya and Claire. Sonya, the stalwart left leg, and Claire, the loose and giddy right one. Sonya might play the role of an exhausted mother or beleaguered elder sister in a Russian black-and-white movie about World War II: a Stakhanovite, doing the work of two all those years and decades.

And Claire? She was a flapper, swinging through life free and easy, never doing any work, just along for the ride. About a decade ago, when I was having circulatory problems in my right leg, a doctor said to me, "I can't promise you're not going to lose that leg," that had seemed perfectly apt: Claire was a gal who might go out for the proverbial pack of cigarettes one night and then—one thing leading to another and then another—get herself lost, never come home.

As for Sonya—she was one of those overburdened women whom middle age hits like a body blow. After doing double duty all these years she sinks into her chair at the end of another hard day and sighs, "I can't believe how tired I am. I'll get up in a minute . . . I can't believe how tired I am. . . . They did an X-ray—bilateral hip, and what do you suppose it showed? Well, frail Claire who's done sweet fuck-all all these years—clean and smooth. Does she show any arthritic changes? Does she? Ha! But me—I've just been worn down by it all. You can see it, right there, in black and white on the X-ray." Sonya might pick up the X-ray, hold it under a visitor's nose, tap the image with her finger over and over again: "See. There's my suffering. Right there. Plain as day. No one can deny it."

When I saw old friends who were postpolio, our conversations began, "Are you doing okay?"

I was more tired than I was when I was twenty; but then again, my nondisabled friends who used to run ten miles a day had started running three.

And then one summer everything fell apart. When I got off a plane in Amsterdam, the heat hit me like a blow to my solar plexus. I must have looked more than just exhausted, I must have looked about to pass out, because people were crowding around, asking if I was all right, to which I answered, "Yes. No." A British voice said, "I say, you're not all right, are you?" The voice came from a plump woman who looked like Miss Marple, with a peaches-and-cream complexion, pure white hair, and a gigantic magnolia blossom sticking out of her carryall. She carried my laptop for me; she took me under her ample wing and shepherded me along to passport control. I was her fledgling, not yet ready to leave the nest. I was her little lost lamb.

"I'll be fine from here," I told her. "Thank you so much. I'm fine. There's my friend. . . . Peter! . . . Thank you."

I said to Peter, "Let's take a cab," and then I was so busy asking Peter how he was and how his partner was and talking about the political situation in the Netherlands and in the world in general, and how I think he will like my friend Celia, that I never got around to telling him about almost fainting when I got off the plane. By the time I got to his apartment on Willemsparkweg, I had allowed myself to forget all about it.

Of course doing what I had done in the past twenty-four hours—taking a taxi from a village in the Sardinian countryside to the train station in Oristano, taking the train from Oristano to Cagliari, sleeping sitting up in a sort of lounge chair on the overnight ferry between Cagliari and Rome, taking the train from where the ferry landed in Rome to Da Vinci Airport and a flight from there to Amsterdam—would have exhausted anybody. But not so much that it seemed they were going to faint when they got off the plane.

But by the end of the summer my muscles were so weak that walking any distance was painful. My son, Max, wanted to play football with me, and I did for a few minutes, in our decidedly unconventional way, and then I lay down on the floor and said, "Honey, I'm too tired. . . . Now we know why the NFL doesn't recruit middle-aged women as players."

When the weather cooled off I got a little better. I cried with happiness the day I had enough energy to wash the kitchen floor.

I was referred to a pulmonologist. Perhaps the cause of my fatigue was respiratory insufficiency. It would be wonderful if it were: A machine would cure me. I imagined myself so filled with energy that I would leap out of bed in the morning singing an ode to the glories of air. At the same time, I hoped it wasn't respiratory insufficiency because I didn't want to lie down every night with a plastic mask over my face attached to a respirator noisily whooshing air in and out of my lungs, beeping when I missed a breath.

Off I went to a pulmonologist, carrying Xeroxes of articles from medical journals that explained late onset postpolio respiratory insufficiency. I remembered all the placating words my freshman comp teacher taught me to avoid, "I think . . . ," "Perhaps . . . ," "I don't know if you . . ." As I handed the pulmonologist my Xeroxed articles, I used all these phrases.

I passed my tests.

No magic bullet.

A couple of winters later, purple splotches appeared on my feet. At first, the doctors thought they were frostbite, probably from a demonstration during which I had sat outside an army recruiting station for two hours in January, to protest the U.S. bombing of Iraq. They turned out to be necrotic tissue. "Necrotic" is derived from a Latin word meaning "dead." The doctor said that I was "throwing" blood clots. (I like medical terminology: not the official Latinate words that appear in charts, but the grim, coarse language medical people use among themselves.) My emergency C-section was called a crash C-section. Dying is coding. "Throwing clots": Sometimes I imagined a girl who looked as if she could have stepped out of an impressionist painting, in a white dress, golden hair with a black ribbon in it, tossing a ball of blood into the air; sometimes I imagined a pitcher hurling a blood ball down one of my veins.)

I asked the vascular specialist, "What's the worst thing that could happen?" because I wanted him to tell me that I wasn't going to die. He said, "I can't promise that you're not going to lose that leg." I had to rush off, the appointment had taken longer than I expected, and Max needed to be picked up at school. Trying to remember what he said was like trying to remember images from a dream. Lose that leg? Did he really say, "lose that leg"? I was upset, but another part of me split off and got goofy: I imagined losing my leg the way I lose my keys and my library card. *Okay, I'm positive I still had my leg when I walked in the door—I mean I walked in the door. I'd have noticed if I was walking in on one leg, wouldn't I?* A novel I read in junior high school about the Civil War, in which there was a field hospital where amputations were performed, came washing up out of my unconscious, where it had been stored away—waiting, I suppose, for just this occasion. I know that if I actually do lose that leg it will not be in a Civil War field hospital with crude saws and buckets of blood and the stink of gangrene: No, it will all be sterile, latex, Plexiglas, white, Demerol (sweet, sweet Demerol!), perfectly unnatural floral arrangements.

When my father was seventy-nine he told me for the first time that he loved me. For years my father had been saying that Sandra, instead of seeing women therapists who didn't have medical degrees, who kept giving her positive reinforcement for the notion that she had been emotionally abused, needed to see a "real" (therefore male) doctor. This doctor would give her medication that would fix her.

My parents went together to the real, male doctor, but the doctor didn't act the way my father had hoped. At Christmastime, when we were home, my father threw himself across the unfolded sofa bed in the study and cried out, "The psychiatrist says it's all my fault! He says it's all my fault! I'm seventy-nine! I'm going to die soon! I love you! He says it's all my fault!"

He sounded like a histrionic actress in a community theater production. I was not in the room, so I don't know what the doctor actually said. But I have spent enough time around the therapeutic professions that I cannot imagine a psychiatrist saying such a thing: I imagine that what the doctor said was, "You have to look at the role you have played," or "You need to examine your own behavior." One of those standard things therapists say when confronted with a family situation in which a family appears, points to one of its members, and says, "We are all fine; everything's fine except for her." But nonetheless my father heard: *It's all your fault.* I am moved by his fragility and by his pain. And at the same time astonished at his emotional immaturity.

Now my son, Max, is nineteen. When he comes home from college he heads off to meet up with his high school friends for a game of slosh softball—you get drunk and then play softball, swinging the bat wildly, stumbling rather than sliding home. "Do you have a designated driver for after the game?" I ask, and hear the answer, "Pretty much." But before he does that, he heads over to see my friend Jenny and her infant son, Jasper. Whenever he calls home, he asks, "How's Jasper?" and I tell him, he's sitting up, he's almost crawling, he's crawling, he's standing. I gave birth to a child who will be the father I longed to have.

When I was in Rhode Island last Christmas, my mother showed me a picture of my father's football team at Winchester High in 1937. "Can you pick out your father?" she asked.

A picture from another world—it's not just that it's in black-and-white, and that the jerseys and trousers are made from wool and cotton, in those prepolyester, prenylon days, but also the all-white school, in contrast to my son's team at Berkeley High, where he is one of a few white faces among the mix of African Americans, Tibetans, Samoans. Those boys of the late 1930s are so much smaller, too—the big bruiser on the team must weigh less than 200 pounds. One day Max called me, wanting to borrow my van, because he was going out with four of his teammates, and when they all got in Max's Chevy, the car was so overloaded the undercarriage dragged on the ground.

"Amy picked him out right away," my mother said. "She said it was easy. He's the one who looks like Max." And sure enough, there is my son's face, staring out at me from a picture taken in 1937.

A SAILBOAT, SAILING INTO THE WIND, TACKS FIRST LEFT, THEN RIGHT, THEN LEFT AGAIN

A few years ago I spent a month at an artists' colony in upstate New York. On one of my last days there, I got in my blue van and drove north, to Saranac Lake. One of the few fragments of memories I have from before I got polio is of sailing on this lake, a week or two before I got sick. The bright orange of the life jackets. The wind in my face. The feel of my mother's arms, holding me tight. A grown-up smiling at me, and me hiding my face against my mother.

I pulled my car over on a crop of land leaning over the lake, and clambered out, leaning on my cane, and sat on a rock, looking out over the water. Beneath me a sailboat, sailing into a headwind, tacked first to the left, glided along for a while, then tacked to the right, sailing catty-corner to the wind. Then to the left again.

I imagined myself as a child on that boat beneath me. Was the virus already incubating within my body? Or only within my mother's body, where it will be a passing intestinal disturbance? There are thousands of imperceptible factors that affect any body's resistance, lack of resistance, to a virus—the acidity of the contents of the stomach, for instance, in the case of a gut virus; whether or not one is fully rested; the individual's mood; one's previous exposure to the virus itself, or to similar viruses. The immune response of a pregnant woman is generally lower, an adaptive response that keeps her body from rejecting the fetus. Change any of those factors—what my mother or I ate for lunch on a certain day, how much sleep we got or did not get on a certain night—and her immune system or mine might have mounted a different response, and the whole course of my life might have changed.

A figure on the boat beneath me—a vague miniature, so distant, I could not tell age or sex or race—manipulated the sail so it luffed and flapped as it caught the wind. A minute difference in the motion of the tiller, an unexpected gust of wind, if not corrected for, sent the sailboat off course: Tiny changes leading to enormous ones.

I tried to imagine that child who is both me and not me, that girl with my genes and my blue eyes and the cowlick at the nape of my neck, clutching at her mother as the sailboat cut across the lake nearly half a century before. And then I tried to imagine that whatever path the virus took from the outer world into first my mother's body and then mine got altered. Imagine my mother in the bathroom of a Gulf station, perhaps on the way back from Saranac Lake that day. Maybe my father is outside, sitting behind the wheel while the gas tank of one of our secondhand green station wagons is getting filled up, or maybe just waiting for her—she has to pee so often, close to the end of her pregnancy. She turns on the hot water rather than the cold, and happens not to touch the faucet that carries a smudge in which the virus teems.

I don't get polio; how do our lives change? My mother wanted to have seven children. It was only when I got sick that she decided to stop at the five she had. So there would have been two other lives in the world. I try to imagine those two younger sisters or two younger brothers—or maybe one of each? What would she have named them? Pam? Cindy? Sally? Tommy? Bill? David? I try to conjure up faces for these ghost sisters and ghost brothers, but when I think "younger sister," I just see Jane's face as a child; "younger brother," and I see John's. At the same time, I have the sensation of missing them, these siblings who existed only as expectations.

A while ago I called my father, and the aide who answers the phone told him, "It's your daughter." "My brother?" my father, who has only a sister, will ask, and I will feel sadness wash over me, for the brother my father never had, for all that my father never had.

I try to factor the disease out of my life, but it's more complicated than the incomprehensible equations I used to proofread at the American Mathematical Society. Probably the two extra children mean even more pressure, financial and otherwise, for my father. Nothing stops his descent into rage and violence. But maybe I don't bear the physical brunt of it. Maybe I'm the one who overhears, safe from behind my closed bedroom door, Cindy or Susan or Jane getting tossed around downstairs; maybe I'm the one who shoves her index fingers into her ears in order not to hear my sister's voice crying out, "Daddy, stop! Please! I'll be good. I promise, I'll be good. Stop!"

Maybe I'm the one who thinks: This is the way I want to live my life, with the door shut tight. Good and tight. Maybe I would have filled the "good daughter" role instead of Susan. I'd be a tenured professor of history or of English. I'd be the one who has never smoked a cigarette or gotten drunk. And since I wouldn't be a taker of risks, and with our family history having a child is taking a risk—childless. So I imagine Max out of existence.

But maybe that sense of defiant willfulness that so enraged my father wasn't something that grew out of my experience—it could have been something fixed and immutable, like the cowlick at the nape of my neck, like my flax-flower-blue eyes. So even without my disability I would still have become one of the targets of his rage. And maybe without that sense of I-can-do-this-I-can-do-anything-quitters-never-win-never-say-die, I would never have survived.

NOTES

THE BARE BONES OF AN ANSWER

"Poliomyelitis is a common . . . ," John R. Paul, *A History of Poliomyelitis* (New Haven: Yale University Press, 1971), p. 1.

"Disease serves . . . ," Charles E. Rosenberg, "Framing Disease: Illness, Society, and History," in *Framing Disease: Studies in Cultural History,* edited by Charles E. Rosenberg and Janet Golden (New Brunswick, N.J.: Rutgers University Press, 1992), p. xviii.

THE STORIES I'M NOT GOING TO TELL

"Every day another muscle . . ." Wilfred Sheed, *In Love with Daylight: A Memoir of Recovery* (New York: Simon and Schuster, 1995), p. 27.

And yet autobiography . . . , David T. Mitchell, "Body Solitaire: The Singular Subject of Disability Autobiography," *American Quarterly* 52(2): 311–15.

Utopians begin by looking in the mirror . . . , Gerald O'Brien, "From Restrictive Marriage to Incentive Provision: Secondary Methods of Eugenic Control." Paper presented at Society for Disability Studies/Canadian Centre on Disability Studies Conference, Winnipeg, June 21, 2001.

A SLIVER OF TIME

"We can now close the book . . . ," quoted in Dorothy Crawford, *The Invisible Enemy: A Natural History of Viruses* (Oxford, England: Oxford University Press, 2000), p. viii. The statement was made in 1969.

PREHISTORY

An ancient Egyptian stele . . . , Dorothy and Philip Sterling, *Polio Pioneers: The Story of the Fight Against Polio* (Garden City, N.Y.: Doubleday, 1955), pp. 8–12.

In the early 1770s Sir Walter . . . , J. G. Lockhart, *Memoirs of Sir Walter Scott*, 1937. http://www.arts.gla.ac.uk/SESLL/stella/STARN/prose/WSCOTT/LIFE/Chap1.htm, retrieved May 24, 2006.

In 1789 the disease . . . , Michael Underwood, *A Treatise on the Diseases of Children with General Directions for the Management of Infants from Birth*, Vol. 2 (London: Mathews, 1789), p. 53.

MYTHS OF ORIGIN

Tracing the origin to somewhere else . . . , Susan Sontag, *AIDS and Its Metaphors* (New York: Farrar, Straus and Giroux, 1988), pp. 17–52.

Early summer in New York . . . , Naomi Rogers, *Dirt and Disease: Polio Before FDR* (New Brunswick, N.J.: Rutgers University Press, 1992), pp. 1–164; Tony Gould, *A Summer Plague: Polio and Its Survivors* (New Haven and London: Yale University Press, 1995), pp. 3–28; Alan M. Kraut, "Plagues and Prejudice: Nativism's Construction of Disease in Nineteenth- and Twentieth-Century New York City," in David Rosner, ed., *Hives of Sickness: Public Health and Epidemics in New York City* (New York: Museum of the City of New York, 1995), pp. 65–90.

A chart showing . . . , *A Monograph on the Epidemic of Poliomyelitis (Infantile Paralysis) in New York City in 1916* (New York: Department of Health of New York City, 1917), n.p.

"Bar all children . . . ," *The New York Times*, July 4, 1916, p. 1.

"25 more deaths . . . ," *The New York Times*, July 5, 1916, p. 1.

"95 more victims . . ." *The New York Times,* July 9, 1916, p. 1.

A newspaper cartoon . . . , *The World* (New York), August 20, 1916, p. 6.

"No doubt many scenes . . . ," George Draper, quoted in Tony Gould, *A Summer Plague: Polio and Its Survivors* (New Haven and London: Yale University Press, 1995), p. 3.

No, before New York . . . , *Infantile Paralysis in Vermont, 1894–1922* (Burlington, Vt.: State Department of Public Health, 1924), pp. 15–68.

And before that . . . , Elisabeth F. Hutchin, "Historical Summary" in *Poliomyelitis; a Survey Made Possible by a Grant from the International Committee for the Study of Infantile Paralysis* (Baltimore: Williams and Wilkins Company, 1932), pp. 1–22.

"Paraplegia set in . . . ," Hippocrates, http://classics.mit.edu/Hippocrates/epidemics/mb.txt, retrieved on August 10, 2004.

"When I was working . . . ," Dorothea Lange, *The Making of a Documentary Photographer*, oral history interview conducted in 1960 and 1961 by Suzanne Riess (Berkeley, Calif.: Regional Oral History Office, Bancroft Library, University of California, Berkeley, 1968), pp. 17–18.

But viruses? . . . , Dorothy Crawford, *The Invisible Enemy*, pp. 5–41.

TELLING SYMPTOMS

In the grip of polio fever . . . , Anne Walters and Jim Marugg, *Beyond Endurance* (New York: Harper and Brothers, 1954), pp. 4–7.

Charles Mee was fourteen . . . , Charles Mee, *A Nearly Normal Life* (Thorndike, Maine: Thorndike Press, 2000) pp. 17–18, 20.

"My brain is a bird . . . ," Lorenzo Milam, *The Cripple Liberation Front Marching Band Blues* (San Diego: Mho and Mho Works, 1984), p. 9.

For Christmas one year . . . , Ernst Doblhofer, *Voices in Stone: The Decipherment of Ancient Scripts and Writings* (New York: Viking Press, 1961), p. 56.

"POLIO STRIKES THE MOST FIT . . . THE MOST BRILLIANT"

When sportswriter Jim Marugg . . . , Walters and Marugg, *Beyond Endurance,* p. 74.

He did such a good job . . . , Bruce Allen Murphy, *Wild Bill: The Legend and Life of William O. Douglas* (New York: Random House, 2003), pp. 282–86.

Roosevelt hid the extent . . . , Hugh Gregory Gallagher, *FDR's Splendid Deception* (New York: Dodd, Mead, 1985), pp. 1–216.

In the mid-1940s . . . , Bentz Plagemann, *My Place to Stand* (New York: Farrar, Straus, 1949), pp. 137, 167.

Peg Kehret, hospitalized in 1949 . . . , Peg Kehret, *Small Steps: The Year I Got Polio* (Morton Grove, Ill.: A. Whitman, 1996), p. 83.

"DO SOMETHING! . . . DO ANYTHING!"

It is hardly surprising . . . , Christopher James Rutty, "Do Something! Do Anything!: Poliomyelitis in Canada, 1927–1962" (Ph.D. thesis, University of Toronto, 1995).

Wanting to help . . . , Hot-wax treatment: Marilyn Rogers's account in Edward J. Sass, with George Gottfried and Anthony Sorem, *Polio's Legacy: An Oral History* (Lanham, Md.: University Press of America, 1996), p. 56; dipping in hot and cold water: telephone interview with Nadina LaSpina, November 21, 2004; rubber mallets: Mary Ann Hoffman in *Polio's Legacy*, p. 137; goose grease: Jack Dominik in *Polio's Legacy*, p. 172; curare injections: Edmund J. Sass's own oral history in *Polio's Legacy*, p. 94.

THE KENNY TREATMENT

"It was such a bizarre, disgusting . . . ," Mee, *A Nearly Normal Life*, pp. 64–65; "Two times every day . . . ," Richard L. Bruno, *The Polio Paradox* (New York: Warner Books, 2002), p. 73.

Sister Kenny wasn't a nun . . . , Elizabeth Kenny with Martha Ostenso, *And They Shall Walk* (New York: Dodd, Mead and Company, 1943); Victor Cohn, *Sister Kenny: The Woman Who Challenged the Doctors* (Minneapolis: University of Minnesota Press, 1976); Wade Alexander, *Sister Elizabeth Kenny: Maverick Heroine of the Polio Treatment Controversy* (Rockhampton, Queensland: Central Queensland University Press, 2003).

"I like to go fast . . . ," Herbert Levine, *I Knew Sister Kenny: A Story of a Great Lady and Little People* (Boston: Christopher Publishing House, 1954), pp. 44–46.

"A person who sapped . . . ," Cohn, *Sister Kenny*, p. 88.

"The clover fields . . . ," Kenny, *And They Shall Walk*, p. 9.

"Two-fisted women called the bush nurses . . . ," *Current Biography: Who's Who and Why*, edited by M. Block (New York: The H. W. Wilson Company, 1942), p. 473.

"At last I tore . . . ," Kenny, *And They Shall Walk*, p. 24.

"The way before you . . . ," Kenny, *And They Shall Walk*, p. 30.

"You have made a great medical discovery . . . ," Levine, *I Knew Sister Kenny*, p. 68.

"I could almost hear . . . ," Noreen Linduska, *My Polio Past* (Chicago: Pellegrini and Cudahy, 1947), p. 59.

"Doctors seeing their patients' twisted necks . . . ," Cohn, *Sister Kenny*, p. 78.

"We did not feel 'sick' . . . ," Edith M. Hall, "In the Ward Next Door to Sister Kenny," *Australian Nurses' Journal* 10, no. 10 (May 1981), pp. 57–58.

Robert C. Huse remembers . . . , Robert C. Huse, *Getting There: Growing Up with Polio in the 30's* (Bloomington, Ind.: 1st Books Library, 2002), pp. 6, 98–99.

Speaking of the atmosphere that prevailed . . . , Nina Gilden Seavey, Jane S. Smith, and Paul Wagner, *A Paralyzing Fear: The Triumph Over Polio in America* (New York: TV Books, 1998), pp. 115–16.

"The nurses were left . . . ," Paul, *A History of Poliomyelitis*, p. 339.

"It boils down to . . . ," Charles H. Andrews, *No Time for Tears* (Garden City, N.Y.: Doubleday and Company, 1952), p. 16.

VARIATIONS ON THE THEME OF VACCINATION
The Polio Pioneers:

"Like a tank driver . . . ," Leonard Kriegel, *Flying Solo: Reimagining Manhood, Courage, and Loss* (Boston: Beacon Press, 1998), p. 34.

In 1952 . . . , "Poliomyelitis: A New Approach," *Lancet*, 1952, 1 (i), p. 552.

"Is all human life equally valuable? . . . ," John Rowan Wilson, *Margin of Safety: The Story of the Poliomyelitis Vaccine* (Garden City, N.Y.: Doubleday and Company, 1963), p. 153.

Thousands upon thousands of people . . . , "Second Annual Vaccine Day Honors Volunteers Nationwide," press release, National Institute of Allergy and Infectious Diseases, National Institutes of Health, May 13, 1999, and "AIDS Vaccine Volunteers Press Their Case," CNN.com, September 25, 1997.

VARIATIONS ON THE THEME OF VACCINATION
The March of Dimes:

There was no end to the hoopla . . . , Gould, *A Summer Plague*, p. 74.

"Fixed with gummy tape . . . ," David W. Rose, *Images of America: March of Dimes* (Charleston, S.C.: Arcadia Publishing, 2004), pp. 9–94.

One picture shows a regiment of women. . . . , http://www.canoe.ca/Lifewise FamilyRetired01/0306_dime_cp.html, retrieved on July 24, 2004.

It wasn't just the swells . . . , "President's Ball to Have Pageant," *The New York Times*, Jan. 21, 1940, p. 40; "Fetes Today Open Fight on Paralysis," *The New York Times*, Jan. 29, 1938, p. 10; "Program at Miami," *The New York Times*, Dec. 29, 1935, p. XX2; and "In one town . . . ," www.clarkstonhistorical .org/newsletters/winter2003 and www.juneauempire.com/stories.

"Victory is imperative . . . ," http://kera.org/tv/productions/fight/default .lasso? Dec. 1, 2004, retrieved on Mar. 19, 2006.

"I could be your child . . . ," "Polio Poster Boy Calls on Truman—Paralysis Foundation Head Lauded," *The New York Times*, Jan. 8, 1952, p. 21; "Polio Poster Baby Wants No Santas," *The New York Times*, Dec. 23, 1949, p. 14.

"Restless belief in the perfectibility . . . ," Wilson, *Margin of Safety*, p. 3.

"Racing for the cure . . . ," Jeff Wise, "Altruism for Fun and Profit," *The New York Times Magazine*, Sept. 7, 1997, p. 64.

VARIATIONS ON THE THEME OF VACCINATION
The Father of Vaccination:

Just as a murkier history . . . , www.fordham.edu/halsall/mod/montagu-smallpox.html, retrieved on May 24, 2006, and http://virus.stanford.edu/pox/history.html, retrieved on May 24, 2006.

"The deviation of man . . . ," Edward Jenner, *An Inquiry into the Causes and Effects of the Variolae Vaccine, or Cow-Pox, 1798,* www.bartelby.com/38/4/1.html, retrieved on May 24, 2006.

VARIATIONS ON THE THEME OF VACCINATION
Polio Vaccine and Aids:

When I spot the book . . . , Edward Hooper, *The River: A Journey to the Source of HIV and AIDS* (Boston, New York, London: Little, Brown and Company, 1999).

VARIATIONS ON THE THEME OF VACCINATION
The End?:

Fears that the polio vaccine . . . , http://news.bbc.co.uk/2/hi/Africa/3513783.stm, retrieved on May 10, 2006.

THERAPY

"It is true that polio . . . ," Andrews, *No Time for Tears,* pp. 144–45.

Leonard Kriegel walked . . . , Leonard Kriegel, *Falling into Life* (San Francisco: North Point Press, 1991), p. 57.

A recent article . . . , Armond S. Goldman, Elisabeth J. Schmalstieg, Daniel H. Freeman, Jr., Daniel A. Goldman, and Frank C. Schmalstieg, Jr., "What Was the Cause of Franklin Delano Roosevelt's Paralytic Illness?" *Journal of Medical Biography* 11 (2003): 232–40.

HOMESICKNESS

The booklets included lists . . . , "Fallout Protection: What to Know and Do About Nuclear Attacks," Department of Defense booklet, Washington, D.C.: Government Printing Office, 1961.

"Nancy Frick recalled . . . ," www.ott.zynet.co.uk/polio/lincolnshire/library/harvest/frick.htm, retrieved on May 24, 2006.

Marilyn Rogers . . . , Wagner, *A Paralyzing Fear*, pp. 27–28.

"They say the sea . . . ," Antonio Gramsci, *Letters from Prison*, Vol. I, edited by Frank Rosengarten, translated by Raymond Rosenthal (New York: Columbia University Press, 1994), p. 229.

I know that sometimes I flipped through . . . , Iris Brooke and James Laver, *English Costume from the Fourteenth Through the Nineteenth Century* (New York: Macmillan Company, 1937), p. 162.

THE MAKINGS OF A DISEASE
The Uses of Illness:

What interests does a disease serve? . . . , Susan Sontag, *Illness As Metaphor* (New York: Farrar, Straus and Giroux, 1978), p. 102; Sontag, p. 70.

THE MAKINGS OF A DISEASE
Made for Each Other:

Dr. Haven Emerson . . . , "Dr. Emerson Dies," *The New York Times*, May 22, 1957, p. 33.

"If the whole *materia medica* . . . ," www.bartleby.com/100/456.html, retrieved July 5, 2006.

By the middle of the nineteenth century . . . , Charles R. King, *Children's Health in America: A History* (New York: Twayne Publishers, 1993), pp. 49–93.

The health authorities did not comprehend . . . , Phyllis H. Williams, *South Italian Folkways in Europe and America: A Handbook for Social Workers, Visiting Nurses, School Teachers, and Physicians* (New York: Russell and Russell, 1969), pp. 170–74.

One nurse, who had been investigating . . . , Ronald Bayer and Amy Fairchild, "The Limits of Privacy: Surveillance and the Control of Disease," *Health Care Analysis* 10, no. 1 (March 2002), pp. 19–35.

Dr. William J. Burns, the health officer of Oyster Bay . . . , G. B. Risse, "Revolt Against Quarantine: Community Responses to the 1916 Polio Epidemic, Oyster Bay, New York," *Transactions and Studies of the College of Physicians of Philadelphia*, 14, no. 1 (Mar. 1992), pp. 23–50.

Italian custom decreed . . . , Williams, *South Italian Folkways in Europe and America*, p. 170.

"In one house I went into . . . ," Al V. Burns, "The Scourge of 1916 . . . America's First and Worst Polio Epidemic," *The American Legion Magazine*, Sept. 1966, p. 45.

THE MAKINGS OF A DISEASE
Overcoming:

In 1875, Jean-Martin Charcot . . . , Richard L. Bruno, *The Polio Paradox: What You Need to Know* (New York: Warner Books, 2002), p. 15; M. Raymond and J. M. Charcot, "Paralysie essentielle de l'enfance, atrophie muscularie consecutive." *Comptes rendus de la Soc de Biology*, 1875, no. 27, p. 158.

"Reports began to surface . . . ," Lauro S. Halstead, "Post-Polio Syndrome," *Scientific American*, 278, no. 4 (April 1998), 36–41.

CRIPPLING GENDER

The year was 1946 . . . , Cohn, *Sister Kenny*, pp. 201–203.

Now that the war was over . . . , Maureen Honey, *Creating Rosie the Riveter: Class, Gender and Propaganda During World War II* (Amherst: University of Massachusetts Press, 1984), pp. 120–26.

"To be tip-toe, dull . . . ," Miriam Dixson, *The Real Matilda: Woman and Identity in Australia, 1788 to the Present* (Sydney: University of New South Wales, 1999), p. 21.

Shortly before shooting . . . , Cohn, *Sister Kenny*, p. 195–96.

Richard Owen was examined by Sister Kenny . . . , Sass, *Polio's Legacy*, p. 34.

As a teenager, Charles Mee . . . , Mee, *A Nearly Normal Life,* pp. 173–76.

An exposé of charities . . . , Ralph Lee Smith, "Canshakers," *True: The Man's Magazine* (Mar. 1963), pp. 41, 80–82.

Charles Mee recalls arriving . . . , Mee, *A Nearly Normal Life,* pp. 13–14.

Edward Le Comte . . . , Edward Le Comte, *The Long Road Back: The Story of My Encounter with Polio* (Boston: Beacon Press, 1957), p. 27.

MARCHING ON THE PENTAGON

Under that headline . . . , Mary Hamilton, "SNCC Leader Asks for Guns," *National Guardian* 19, no. 49 (September 9, 1967), p. 5.

The *Guardian* posed the question . . . , "White Radicals Respond to Ghetto Rebellion," 19, no. 48 (September 2, 1967), p. 4.

The *National Guardian* also ran a full-page ad . . . , *National Guardian* 19, no. 40 (July 8, 1967), p. 9.

"Asthma is threatening me seriously . . . ," Ernesto Guevara, *Che's Diary* (Nottingham, England: Bertrand Russell Peace Foundation, 1968), pp. 139, 140, 164.

About ten days before . . . , "McNamara Heckled As War Critics Halt His Car at Harvard," *The New York Times,* Nov. 8, 1966, p. 1.

General Wheeler . . . , "Students and Police Clash at Pembroke As Wheeler Speaks," *The New York Times,* Nov. 16, 1966, p. 5.

Do I still have . . . , Felix Greene, *Vietnam! Vietnam!* (Palo Alto, Calif.: Fulton Publishing Company, 1966), pp. 45, 79.

SCHOOL HOUSE CANDY

And I had read . . . , *John Dos Passos, 1919* (New York: Harcourt, Brace and Company, 1932), pp. 105–106.

In his seminal essay . . . , Randolph Bourne, "The Handicapped," *Atlantic Monthly* (September 1911), pp. 320–29.

"Had I read of Jacobus tenBroek . . . , Jacobus tenBroek and Floyd Matson, *Hope Deferred: Public Welfare and the Blind* (Berkeley: University of California Press, 1959).

In New York in the 1930s . . . , Paul K. Longmore and David Goldberger, "The League of the Physically Handicapped and the Great Depression: A Case Study in the New Disability History," in Longmore's *Why I Burned My Book and Other Essays on Disability* (Philadelphia: Temple University Press, 2003), pp. 53–101.

People with disabilities also gained entry into the workforce . . . , Huse, pp. 206, 210.

HUMPTY-DUMPTY

"All available evidence . . . ," Bruno, *The Polio Paradox*, p. 20.

This shift is illustrated . . . , Alan Marshall, *I Can Jump Puddles* (Melbourne, Australia: F. W. Cheshire, 1955), p. 2.

Eleanor Roosevelt . . . , http://www.uusociety.org/sermons/first_lady_10_19_ 03.html, retrieved on May 14, 2006.

The murder of fourteen-year-old Emmett Till . . . , *The Tavis Smiley Show,* NPR, broadcast November 14, 2002.

Another direct link . . . , Corbett O'Toole, *Corbett O'Toole* (Berkeley, Calif.: (Regional Oral History Office, University of California Berkeley, 1998), http://ark.cdlib.org/ark:/13030/kt4779n6sq.